Q
50

D1188627

Writing Health Communication

WITHDRAWN

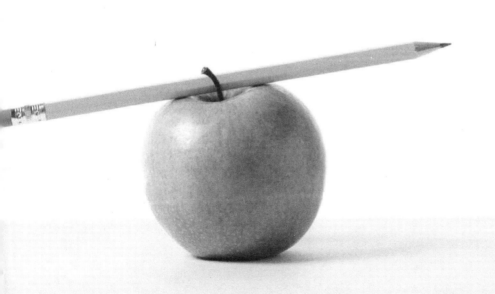

SAGE has been part of the global academic community
since 1965, supporting high quality research and learning
that transforms society and our understanding of individuals,
groups, and cultures. SAGE is the independent, innovative,
natural home for authors, editors and societies who share
our commitment and passion for the social sciences.

Find out more at: **www.sagepublications.com**

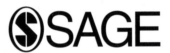

Writing Health Communication

An Evidence-based Guide

Charles Abraham and Marieke Kools

NORTH HAMPSHIRE HOSPITAL HEALTHCARE LIBRARY

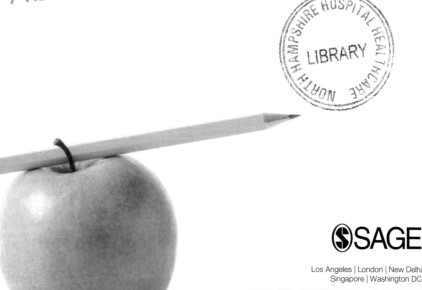

$SAGE

Los Angeles | London | New Delhi
Singapore | Washington DC

Chapter 1 © Marieke Kools and Charles Abraham 2012
Chapter 2 © James Hartley 2012
Chapters 3 and 4 © Marieke Kools
Chapter 5 © Pat Wright 2012
Chapter 6 and 7 © Charles Abraham 2012

Chapter 8 © Rob Ruiter and Gerjo Kok 2012
Chapter 9 © Marieke Werrij, Rob Ruiter, Jonathan van 't Reit and Heinde Vries 2012
Chapter 10 © Hans Brug and Anke Oenema 2012
Chapter 11 © Charles Abraham and Marieke Kools 2012

First published 2012

Apart from any fair dealing for the purposes of research or private study, or criticism or review, as permitted under the Copyright, Designs and Patents Act, 1988, this publication may be reproduced, stored or transmitted in any form, or by any means, only with the prior permission in writing of the publishers, or in the case of reprographic reproduction, in accordance with the terms of licences issued by the Copyright Licensing Agency. Enquiries concerning reproduction outside those terms should be sent to the publishers.

SAGE Publications Ltd
1 Oliver's Yard
55 City Road
London EC1Y 1SP

SAGE Publications Inc.
2455 Teller Road
Thousand Oaks, California 91320

SAGE Publications India Pvt Ltd
B 1/I 1 Mohan Cooperative Industrial Area
Mathura Road
New Delhi 110 044

SAGE Publications Asia-Pacific Pte Ltd
3 Church Street
#10-04 Samsung Hub
Singapore 049483

Library of Congress Control Number: 2011929697

British Library Cataloguing in Publication data

A catalogue record for this book is available from the British Library

ISBN 978-1-84787-185-5
ISBN 978-1-84787-186-2 (pbk)

Typeset by C&M Digitals (P) Ltd, India, Chennai
Printed by MPG Books Group, Bodmin, Cornwall
Printed on paper from sustainable resources

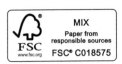

Dedication

It was during work with Professor Herman Schaalma (1959–2009) at Maastricht University that Charles Abraham and Marieke Kools met and began to discuss this book. Herman spent his career working tirelessly to evaluate and improve health promotion practice. He encouraged work on this book and would have loved to have seen it in print. Sadly, he died before the project was completed. We dedicate this book to his memory.

Contents

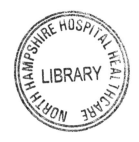

NORTH HAMPSHIRE HOSPITAL HEALTHCARE LIBRARY

Contents

Detailed contents

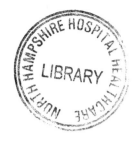

NORTH HAMPSHIRE HOSPITAL
HEALTHCARE
LIBRARY

Detailed contents

Detailed contents

Detailed contents

About the editors

Charles Abraham is Professor of Behaviour Change in the Peninsula College of Medicine & Dentistry at the University of Exeter, UK. He conducts research into health promotion and sustainable energy use, and studies motivational and volitional processes that regulate action. His research focuses on developing and evaluating behaviour change interventions. Charles also provides training, consultancy and policy advice. Charles is a visiting professor at the Universities of Sussex, Nottingham and Maastricht, and a Research Associate at the Center for Health, Intervention, and Prevention (CHIP) at the University of Connecticut. He has been co-editor of the journal *Psychology and Health* and was the founding chair of the British Psychological Society, Division of Health Psychology. Charles has also worked as a research consultant to the Department of Health in the UK. He was a member of the National Institute for Health and Clinical Excellence (NICE) group which developed the 2007 guidelines on Behaviour Change practice and was Specialist Advisor to the House of Lords Select Committee on Science and Technology inquiry into Behaviour Change in 2011.

(http://www.pcmd.ac.uk/profiles.php?id= cabraham&tab=full).

Marieke Kools is a behavioural scientist at the Faculty of Health, Medicine and Life Sciences at Maastricht University in the Netherlands. With a background in experimental cognitive psychology (cognitive educational psychology as well as cognitive ergonomics), her research focuses on the usability of written information, with a specific interest in health education materials. Central in her applied experimental studies is the question of how layout and design characteristics can influence message comprehension and attention processes in readers. Marieke uses existing health education brochure materials to assess effects of textual as well as graphical design elements on how readers use and understand these materials. Marieke also provides training and consultancy regarding the design and evaluation of health promotion materials. She recently shifted her focus towards teaching and coaching medical doctors at the Institute of General Practitioners Education at Maastricht University.

(email: Marieke.kools@maastrichtuniversity.nl)

About the contributors

Johannes Brug is Professor of Epidemiology and Director of the EMGO Institute for Health and Care Research at the VU University Medical Center, Amsterdam, in the Netherlands. Johannes's main research interests are in the development and evaluation of health education and health promotion interventions, with a special interest in behavioural nutrition and physical activity. His research covers studies on the determinants of health behaviours, small-scale experimentation with innovative health education interventions, and larger-scale field experiments in which the efficacy and external validity of health-promoting interventions are evaluated.

(http://www.emgo.nl/personal_pages/profile/index.asp?id=476&page=1)

Hein de Vries is Professor of Health Communication at Maastricht University in the Netherlands. He has a strong interest in theories and theory development on psycho-social determinants of health behaviour, in particular, attitudes, social influences and self-efficacy; planning models for health promotion and health psychology; and development, evaluation and diffusion of interventions (e.g. video-peer-led programmes, school programmes, work site programmes, self-help manuals, computer tailoring).

(http://www.personeel.unimaas.nl/hein.devries/Default.htm)

James Hartley is Honorary Research Professor of Psychology at the University of Keele, Staffordshire, UK. His main research interests lie in written communication, with especial reference to typography and layout, but he is also well known for his research into teaching and learning in the context of higher education. Professor Hartley is a Fellow of both the British Psychological Society and the American Psychological Association. He has published a series of books including *Designing Instructional Text*, 3rd edition (Kogan Page, 1994) and *Academic Writing and Publishing: A Practical Handbook* (Routledge, 2008) (email: j.hartley@psy.keele.ac.uk)

(http://www.keele.ac.uk/depts/ps/people/jhartley/index.htm)

Gerjo Kok is former Dean and Professor of Applied Psychology at the Faculty of Psychology and Neuroscience at Maastricht University. He held the Dutch AIDS Fund endowed professorship for AIDS prevention and health promotion, 1992–2004. His main research interests are the application of social psychology to health promoting behaviour, energy conservation, traffic safety, and the prevention of stigmatisation.

(http://www.psychology.unimaas.nl/Base/Medewerkerspersonal/GerjoKok_extended.htm)

Anke Oenema is Associate Professor of Health Communication in the Department of Health Promotion at Maastricht University in the Netherlands. Her main research interests are in development, evaluation and innovation of computer-tailored interventions aimed at the promotion of dietary and physical activity behaviours and obesity prevention. She focuses on improving efficacy and reach of interventions by delivering computer-tailored interventions through new media, to implement 'new' variables such as environmental factors, and on applying new techniques such as motivational interviewing in computer-tailored programs.

(http://survey.erasmusmc.nl/intern/pwp/?aoenema)

Rob Ruiter is Associate Professor of Applied Psychology at Maastricht University in the Netherlands. His research focuses on studying the effects of persuasive health messages and the underlying change mechanisms. He also has a strong interest in research capacity building in Sub-Saharan Africa through developing and testing theory- and evidence-based health promotion interventions while training young students to become fully qualified public health researchers.

(http://ruiter.socialpsychology.org)

Jonathan van 't Riet is a Researcher at Wageningen University and Research Center. His research interests are in consumer behaviour. He specialises in the determinants of food choice and the effects of health communication messages, with a special interest in message framing and defensive reactions to health-promoting messages.

Marieke Werrij is a Lecturer in the Department of Occupational Therapy of Zuyd University of Applied Sciences in the Netherlands. Marieke previously worked as a researcher in the field of health promotion at Maastricht University. Her main research interests are persuasive communication, with a special interest in message framing, and the cognitive approach to (the treatment of) obesity.

Patricia Wright is Professor Emerita at the School of Psychology, Cardiff University, Wales. Patricia is a Fellow of the British Psychological Society. Her research explores how the design of information influences people's behaviour with printed and online materials. (email: wrightp1@cardiff.ac.uk)

1

Introduction: steps towards writing effective educational text

Marieke Kools and Charles Abraham

Healthcare professionals are regularly involved in creating and commissioning a range of written health education materials including patient information sheets and leaflets promoting health-related behaviours. Increasingly, these materials include electronic formats, including websites. The purpose of such materials may be to inform people about health, medicines, medical products or medical procedures or to persuade people to make healthy choices and help them to change health-related behaviour patterns.

1.1 Are written health education and promotion materials evidence-based?

Research suggests that there is a gap between evidence and practice in the development of health promotion materials: the presentation and message content of health promotion materials do not appear to follow evidence-based best practice. For example, Coulter et al. (1999) found that patient information leaflets do not generally provide the information that patients want and, in a national UK survey, Payne et al. (2000) found that only 40 per cent of the population would be able to understand leaflets produced by UK palliative care units. This lack of correspondence between content and presentation and research findings means that, at best, these materials are *less* likely to: (1) engage their intended audience; (2) meet readers' informational needs; (3) enhance readers' motivation; and (4) provide readers with the skills necessary to act on their motivation. At worst, this may mean that written materials may not be read and, when read, may have no beneficial effects. Ineffective materials are also cost ineffective; they represent a waste of effort and investment for both the authors and the audience. Research has shown that the form and layout of health education materials greatly affect readers' motivation to read, and the ease with which readers engage with and understand, the written materials. Yet many health-promoting written texts fail to employ effective presentation techniques. Educational and persuasive materials are also much more likely to instigate change if their content is carefully matched to the needs and readiness-to-change of their target audience. Achieving this match requires careful planning. Detailed step-by-step guidance on how to achieve such matching is available. Yet, the content of health promotion materials often does not reflect such advice.

1.2 Aims of this book

This book maps out research-based recommendations for improving educational and persuasive texts so that they impact on readers' attention, comprehension, motivation and behavioural skills. We will summarise current evidence on how to make such materials accessible and effective. Whether you are writing or commissioning health education materials or are otherwise involved in developing persuasive written materials, this book will help you make the right choices to reach your audience and help them change their behaviour.

We have emphasised practical, evidence-based guidance. Consequently, we have not provided complete reference lists but included only references to research essential to understanding points made in each chapter. The research referenced here will guide curious readers towards a wider research literature.

1.3 Reading this book

The chapters in this book are set out so that the early chapters focus on layout and presentation while the later chapters focus on message contents. Each chapter can be read on its own, although we do recommend that you read Chapter 6 before Chapter 7. You may dip into the book, depending on your design goals and questions and the design stage you have reached. Each chapter is carefully structured so, using the detailed contents pages, you can quickly find sections you have read before. *Chapter 11* by Abraham and Kools provides a summary of the key insights and recommendations, so one effective way of using the book is to read Chapter 11 first. This will highlight the key ideas which you can then follow up in detail by reading the preceding chapters.

To make the content accessible, each chapter starts with a short list of 'learning outcomes'. Reading this first you can scan through the chapter headings to understand the structure before you start reading. You may find you want to read the chapter in a different order to that set out by the author, depending on what you really want to know.

1.4 The design process and the book structure

This book has two main areas of focus, corresponding to two essential considerations when designing health promotion materials, namely: 'How should we present the information?' and 'How should the message contents be designed?'. So, both the format and content of the message are discussed. Each chapter sets out the choices you need to make to develop effective materials. We have presented the chapter content in a practical manner focusing on what you need to do to improve your written materials. Each chapter uses concrete examples and provides guidance and tips on how to effectively incorporate evidence-based features. Throughout the book we stress that the design process is iterative – you as a health promotion specialist make choices related to the content and layout of your materials, involve representatives of your target audience to pre-test and test your designs, and, based on the feedback you receive, adjust your materials, seek further feedback and so on. Specifically, we propose the following design cycle, including several stages in which different questions need to be answered:

Stage 1 Design the basic layout

What constraints do different kinds of leaflets or brochures impose on the text design? In practice, this is often not a real 'choice', since many public health organisations responsible for the publication of health promotion materials have their own standard print and website format or house style that health promoters need to use. However, even then, or we would argue *especially* then, we advise you to look critically at this format and discuss the elements you feel need to change to prevent adverse effects on your readers. *Chapter 2* by Hartley describes basic text elements such as page size, line spacing and text margins, and their effects on readers.

Stage 2 Use text structure, graphics and colour to maximise attention, accessibility and impact

Funding may be an important enabling or restricting factor determining choices for additional layout features such as the use of graphics in the form of illustrations, pictures, icons, and the use of colour. Chapters 3–5 focus on these issues from different perspectives. Although these early chapters focus on presentational issues, in fact, these issues may become more important once you have decided on content (the focus of Chapters 6–10). Once a first draft of your health promotion text has been developed, including ideas for supporting graphics, it is important to take a step back and have a critical look at it. Having focused thus far on the contents of your materials, it is now important to make sure that the text will engage readers' attention and that they will understand it – otherwise carefully planned content may have no effect on readers.

A key question for designers at this stage is: 'Will my target audience understand my messages?' Whereas in the previous stages of the design cycle, you kept your target audience in mind regarding *what* messages will persuade them, now you need to consider *how* to best put those messages across. *Chapter 3* by Kools draws upon research in cognitive psychology to explain how people generally process information, and what implications this has for health promotion text design. The chapter invites you to adopt specific design approaches to text elements you want readers to pay most attention to, those which only need to be understood and those that need to be remembered, or acted upon.

Chapter 4 by Kools takes a further step and, applying a cognitive ergonomical perspective, describes how to design and evaluate for maximal usability. The chapter discusses how to make your materials optimally accessible for different readers with different goals. This ergonomical approach introduces a new, helpful way of thinking about designing health promotion texts. *Chapter 5* by Wright focuses on the use of graphics and provides a guide as to how to maximise the impact and utility of graphics for readers. This chapter highlights challenges involved in using graphics and provides an evidence-based approach to avoiding pitfalls. Note that Chapter 3 also provides additional insights that may help you choose the best supporting graphics and evaluate both textual and graphical elements in relation to how easily they can be understood by readers. Again these chapters emphasise the importance of pre-testing materials with small groups of target readers.

Stage 3 Get the message right

Most designers of health promotion texts begin with a clear view of what they want to communicate to their audience. For example, if the problem is transmission of infection, the solution may be to tell readers to wash their hands. Alternatively, if the problem is that young people drink too much alcohol, the solution is to tell them how to drink less. It may appear that 'getting the message right' is just a matter of common sense. Designers may conclude that the main work is to ensure good pre-sentation and layout (as covered in Chapters 2–5). In fact, getting the message right is not easy. Recently we watched a research presentation by Joanne Smith of Exeter University, UK (Smith et al., in preparation) that illustrates this point clearly. Joanne tested the effects of a campaign designed to reduce binge drinking among students. Using an experimental design in laboratory conditions, she found that, compared to students who were not exposed to the campaign, those who saw the campaign had stronger intentions to binge drink. These results imply that the campaign, which had already been launched, was encouraging binge drinking. Although the campaign advised against binge drinking, it also gave the impression that most students were binge drinking and enjoying it. These implicit messages motivated other students to binge drink. So common-sense approaches do not necessarily generate effective health promotion. Fortunately, there is a substantial and informative body of research on how to design messages that effectively change motivation and behaviour. Chapters 6–10 present this research in an accessible and practical format.

Chapter 6 by Abraham uses two integrative theoretical frameworks based on a wide range of studies to identify key change targets when trying to promote motivation and behaviour change. This chapter illustrates how the designer can select evidence-based change targets and can precisely match message content to those targets. Chapter 6 also emphasises how important it is know what the target audience believe and, in general, how ready they are to change. *Chapter 7* by Abraham builds on the ideas presented in Chapter 6. Drawing on a wider body of research, this chapter considers the new change targets that are important when seeking to change motivation and behaviour. The chapter shows how for each change target, a variety of change techniques can be employed – and again emphasises how knowing the target audience can help select the most appropriate technique. A menu of 40 behaviour change techniques is presented and discussed. As in other chapters the role of planning and evaluation is emphasised.

Chapter 8 by Ruiter and Kok considers in detail one particular approach to behaviour change, namely emphasising the severity of consequences following from risky behaviour patterns, and frightening people regarding their own actions. This chapter acknowledges such fear arousal is popular among health promoters but also draws upon a large body of research to show that fear arousal may have counter-productive effects because people defend themselves against frightening messages. The chapter explains how to design effective fear appeals but also recommends that designers consider other behaviour change techniques.

Chapter 9 by Werrij, Ruiter, van 't Riet and de Vries demonstrates that even when the content of health promotion messages has been carefully considered, the exact formulation – or framing – of those messages can determine their effectiveness. Different target behaviours may require different message wording. These subtle but important effects are often overlooked by health promoters. This chapter explains the evidence and makes clear recommendations for practice.

Chapter 10 by Brug and Oenema acknowledges the opportunities that electronic media offer health promoters. The chapter discusses the construction and evaluation of computer-tailored interventions. Such interventions have the capacity to shape – or tailor – messages – not to the target group – but to the individual reader. While construction of these systems is more time-consuming and expensive, they may be more cost effective if shown to be more effective than paper-based messages. This chapter considers the relevant evidence and guides designers through the construction of computer-tailored interventions.

Stage 4 Test the effectiveness of the intervention

This design stage may be the most crucial and at the same time most neglected. A designer may have made good choices and implemented appropriate behaviour change techniques in a manner that optimises comprehension and usability, yet it remains an empirical question as to whether the final product is effective. Throughout this book we illustrate how evaluations can feed back into good design. Involving members of the target audience is crucial: only then can valid predictions regarding the effects of your interventions can be made. We would like to stress here that a focus on contents as well as layout in this testing phase is important to give you a complete picture of both these aspects of effective health promotion design. Designers need to discover how people use their materials, i.e., what information they are looking for, what will stand out for them, what they will understand and remember and what effect reading the materials will have on their motivation and behaviour. Findings from pre-tests and full evaluations can be used to make well-founded changes to original designs, thus continuing an iterative process that is likely to maximise effectiveness. Evaluations also provide invaluable guidance for the development of future materials.

Note

The work was partially supported by the National Institute for Health Research (NIHR) UK. However, the views expressed are those of the authors and not necessarily those of the NIHR or the UK Department of Health.

References

Abraham, C (2011a) 'Developing evidence-based content for health promotion materials', in C. Abraham, and M. Kools (eds), *Writing Health Communication: An Evidence-Based Guide*. London: Sage.

Abraham, C (2011b) 'Mapping change mechanisms on to behaviour change techniques: a systematic approach to promoting behaviour change through text', in C. Abraham, and M. Kools (eds), *Writing Health Communication: An Evidence-Based Guide*. London: Sage.

Abraham, C. and Kools, M. (2011) 'Conclusions and recommendations', in C. Abraham, and M. Kools (eds), *Writing Health Communication: An Evidence-Based Guide*. London: Sage.

Brug, H. And Oenema, A. (2011) 'Computer-tailoring of health promotion messages', in C. Abraham, and M. Kools (eds), *Writing Health Communication: An Evidence-Based Guide*. London: Sage.

Coulter, A., Entwistle, V. and Gilbert, D. (1999) 'Sharing decisions with patients: is the information good enough?' *British Medical Journal*, 318: 318–22.

Hartley, J. (2011) 'Designing easy-to-read text', in C. Abraham, and M. Kools (eds), *Writing Health Communication: An Evidence-Based Guide*. London: Sage.

Kools, M. (2011a) 'Making written materials easy to understand', in C. Abraham, and M. Kools (eds), *Writing Health Communication: An Evidence-Based Guide*. London: Sage.

Kools, M. (2011b) 'Making written materials easy to use', in C. Abraham, and M. Kools (eds), *Writing Health Communication: An Evidence-Based Guide*. London: Sage.

Payne, S., Large, S., Jarrett, N. and Turner, P. (2000) 'Written information given to patients and families by palliative care units: a national survey', *The Lancet*, 355: 1792.

Ruiter, R. and Kok, G. (2011) 'Planning to frighten people? Think again!', in C. Abraham, and M. Kools (eds), *Writing Health Communication: An Evidence-Based Guide*. London: Sage.

Smith, J.R., Louis, W.R. and Terry, D.J. (in preparation) 'When norms backfire: descriptive norm inferences can undermine injunctive norm effects'.

Werrij, M., Ruiter, R., van 't Riet, J. and de Vries, H. (2011) 'Message framing', in C. Abraham, and M. Kools (eds), *Writing Health Communication: An Evidence-Based Guide*. London: Sage.

Wright , P. (2011) 'Using graphics effectively in text', in C. Abraham, and M. Kools (eds), *Writing Health Communication: An Evidence-Based Guide*. London: Sage.

2

Designing easy-to-read text

James Hartley

If text is to be persuasive, it must be read. If it is not easy to read, then it will be ignored or misunderstood. In this chapter I focus, not on the content of the text, but on how to arrange the text so that it is easier to read. In particular, I discuss the layout and typographical design of health promotion and medical information, and I provide guidelines that are applicable to posters, books, leaflets and screen-based presentations.

Learning Outcomes

After reading this chapter, you should be able to:

1 List and consider the factors that are important in choosing a page size and page orientation.
2 Use consistent spacing around a text to optimise understanding.
3 Use the most appropriate type-sizes and typefaces.
4 Use devices to emphasise and differentiate text sparingly and carefully (e.g., italic, bold, underlining, capital letters, and colour).

First, come with me into my doctor's waiting room and look around. There are several written notices on the walls. The majority of these are colourful professional posters on various topics such as smoking and travel care. Most of these I cannot read from where I am sitting because the print is too small or it is too pale. I *can* see, however, that the travel care leaflet says (two-thirds of the way down) 'Going Abroad? Things You Need To Know', but I would have to get up and go closer to it to find out what these things are. On other walls there are hand-written and word-processed notices. Again, none of these can be read clearly from where I am sitting, nor from any other seats. They are too small, they use a lot of capital letters, and they are badly spaced.

Most waiting rooms are like this – some better, some worse. In hospitals, for instance, the walls of waiting areas are often crowded with leaflets and hand-produced posters forbidding this and encouraging that. Generally speaking, they are all badly produced. What is wrong with these materials? What can we do to improve them?

2.1 Choosing page sizes and orientations

Printed texts come in all shapes and sizes. There are no specific rules that might suggest to writers, designers or printers why they should choose one particular size in preference to another. The research literature on information design offers little help, for page size is not an issue featured in many books on this topic. Yet the choice of page size constrains all of the subsequent decisions. We cannot discuss column widths, line lengths, type sizes and typefaces until we know the size of the page on which the text will be printed. It is the size of the page (and screen) that determines the size of the overall visual display. The reader needs to be able to scan, read, and focus on both gross and fine details in this display. A number of factors contribute to decisions about which page size to employ. Perhaps the most important of these is how the text is going to be used. Other factors are reader preferences and expectations, particular design features (e.g., when leaflets are to be folded to fit in the packaging), and the costs of production and marketing.

2.1.1 Standard page sizes

The page sizes that we commonly see are cut from much larger basic printing sheets that have been folded several times. The great variety in these page sizes comes from manufacturers using different sizes for their basic printing sheets and then folding them in different ways.

In 1911, Wilhelm Oswald proposed the ratio 1:1.414 (that is, 1:$\sqrt{2}$) as the 'world format'. Then, in 1922, the German standard, DIN 476, was published. Here the ratio of width:height as 1:$\sqrt{2}$ was retained with a basic printing sheet size of one square metre. The International Organisation for Standardisation (ISO) adopted this standard in 1958, together with the A, B and C series of sizes. Today the 50 or more national standards bodies that make up the ISO recommend this series.

The ISO series is widely used in Europe, especially the A4 and A5 sizes (297 x 210 mm and 210 x 148mm). The unifying principle of the ISO-recommended sizes is that a rectangle with sides in the ratio of 1:$\sqrt{2}$ can be halved or doubled to produce a series of rectangles, each of which retains the proportions of the original. A rectangle of any other proportion will generate geometrically similar rectangles only at every other point in the process of halving or doubling. Try folding an A4 and other-sized sheets in half and you will see how this works.

As the pages of a book are made by folding the larger basic printing sheet in half – once, twice, three or more times – all of the pages made from an ISO standard size basic sheet will be in the ratio of 1:$\sqrt{2}$. Sheets that do not follow this standard are not geometrically similar when folded, and this creates waste.

Pages, of course, can be bound in a vertical (*portrait*) or a horizontal (*landscape*) style. (Turn this book on its side to judge the effect.) Pages can be also be bound at the top (as in a notebook) as well as on the left. These variations allow for a variety of page layouts within the different orientations (see Hartley, 2004a). Curiously enough, there is almost no research comparing the effects of setting the same text *portrait* or *landscape*. The only study that I do know of in this respect compared a simulated printed patient information leaflet presented in both orientations (Hartley and Johnson, 2000). Table 2.1 shows how page size and orientation interacts with and controls a number of subsequent decisions. A landscape orientation, for example, facilitates the use of multiple columns.

Table 2.1   The typographic features of patient information leaflets (Data percentages based on a sample of 100 leaflets.)

	Portrait style (75% of the sample) (%)	Landscape style (25% of the sample) (%)
1 column	48	0
2 columns	50	83
3 columns	2	5
4 columns	0	10
5 columns +	0	2
justified text	74	62
unjustified text	26	38
left-ranging headings	86	65
centred headings	14	35
headings in lower-case	82	48
headings in capitals	18	52
diagrams included	16	35
no diagrams	84	65
photos included	10	8
no photos	90	92
boxed in text	10	15
no boxed in text	90	85

2.1.2 Margins

In many books (and leaflets) there are equally wide margins at the top, bottom and sides. In some cases the space devoted to the margins in this way can occupy up to 50 per cent of the page. In practice, however, a margin of about 10mm is necessary at the top, bottom and outer margins of the page, but the inner, or binding edge, margin is a special case. Here we need to consider factors that suggest the need for a wider margin. For example, the printed page may be copied at some time, and the copies punched or clipped for filing with other material. The binding system itself may involve the punching of pages, or it may be such that text or diagrams printed too close to the binding edge curve inwards and are difficult to read (or to copy). So, since text often appears on both the front and

Designing easy-to-read text

the back of a page, a margin of about 25mm is necessary for both the inner left-and the inner right-hand margins.

2.1.3 Column widths

The choice of column widths depends upon the size and orientation of the page, the widths of the margins, and the nature of the text. As seen in Table 2.1, printed leaflets set landscape were more likely to use a double or multiple-column format. Other variations, such as one wide column and one narrow one, are possible, and it is useful to consider these when planning the size and positioning of tables, figures, and other such illustrative materials. Magazines tend to vary their column formats from one page to the next for different kinds of text, but this might be confusing for readers of more serious materials. Screen-based text, too, often uses more than a single-column.

2.2 Spacing text

The way space is organised affects how easy it is for the reader to understand and retrieve the information from it. Thus the clarity of the text can be enhanced by a rational and consistent use of the 'white space'.

Small (1997) points out that books began originally as vertical rolls when the concept of a page did not exist, and there were no page breaks or page numbers. In Classical Greek times, there were no breaks between words, sentences or even paragraphs. (The paragraph as a unit of text on the page did not appear until the sixteenth century.) Cross-references were vague, like 'see above' and 'see below'. The letters forming the words were of the same height, and often of the same width. Line lengths were equal, and words were split at the ends of lines without hyphenation. Figure 2.1 shows what such text would look like if it were printed but, of course, such texts were handwritten. Today, punctuation and spacing, together with upper and lower-case letters, make text easier to read. And so does spacing between paragraphs, sub-sections and chapters.

Evidence from eye-movement research suggests that these spatial arrangements provide important cues for understanding text. Fisher (1976), for instance,

```
FORADULTSANDCHILDRENOVER12TAKE10R2TABL
ETSWITHFOOD20R3TIMESADAYDONOTTAKEMORE
THAN6TABLETSINTWENTYFOURHOURSLEAVEATL
EAST4HOURSBETWEENDOSESDONOTGIVETHISM
EDICINETOCHILDRENUNDER12DONOTTAKETHISM
EDICINEDURINGPREGNANCYITMAYDELAYLABOUR
ORMAKEITLASTLONGER
```

Figure 2.1   A schematic presentation of classical Greek text

Writing health communication

argues that with increasing maturity and experience, readers come to rely more heavily on such cues to enhance their reading and search efficiency. Research has also shown that the beginning of a line – and not its end – has a more marked effect on eye-movement fixations, and also that text that starts in an irregular manner, such as poetry, produces more looking back (regressive fixations) than does regularly spaced text.

Consistent and systematic spacing helps the reader:

1   to see the structure of the document as a whole;
2   to see redundancies in the text, and thus enables him or her to read faster;
3   to see more easily which bits of the text are personally relevant.

Accordingly, text designers should employ systematic spacing, rather than altering the spacing for aesthetic reasons as the text proceeds.

2.2.1 Vertical spacing

Spacing can be considered both vertically and horizontally. The underlying structure of complex text can be made more apparent to the reader by a consistent and pre-planned use of vertical spacing. In practice, this means that pre-determined increments of line-space can be used consistently throughout the text to separate the sub-components – such as sentences, paragraphs, sub- and major headings.

One simple way of using line-space in this way is to use it in a proportional system. One can, for example, separate paragraphs by one line-space; separate sub-headings from paragraphs by two extra lines above and one below them; and separate main headings from text or sub-headings by four extra lines above and two below them. With more complex text one can even start each sentence on a new line within each paragraph.

The top part of Figure 2.2 shows a traditionally spaced piece of text, and the bottom part a revised version of it using a systematic spacing system. Such a system provides an effective way of determining that the amount of space between the component parts of a piece of text is consistent throughout the work. Other systems (not necessarily proportional, but nonetheless consistent) can be used. Indeed, for even more complex text, one might wish to introduce indentation into the text to convey further substructure (as we shall see below).

Research has shown that readers usually prefer lengthy paragraphs to be printed in this more open manner both in print and on screen (Hartley, 2004a; Ling and van Schaik, 2007). Thus readers generally prefer text set in the bottom arrangement shown in Figure 2.2.

Finally, in relation to vertical spacing, we need to note that if the vertical spacing between the components of the text is consistent throughout the text, then this will lead to text with a 'floating baseline'. This means that, in contrast to most textbooks – including this one – the text will not always finish at the same place on every page, irrespective of its content. With a floating baseline the stopping

Designing easy-to-read text

For adults and children over 12 take 1 or 2 tablets with food 2 or 3 times a day. Do not take more than 6 tablets in 24 hours. Leave at least 4 hours between doses. Do not give this medicine to children under 12. Do not take this medicine during pregnancy. It may delay labour or make it last longer.

For adults and children over 12

Take 1 or 2 tablets with food 2 or 3 times a day.

Do not take more than 6 tablets in 24 hours.

Leave at least 4 hours between doses.

Do not give this medicine to children under 12.

Do not take this medicine during pregnancy.
It may delay labour or make it last longer.

Figure 2.2   Top: text set in a traditional layout; bottom: text set with consistent vertical spacing

point for each page is determined by the content and the structure of the text rather than by the need to fill the page.

As a rule of thumb we can say that each page in a printed textbook (or a screen or leaflet) should have a specified number of lines, plus or minus two. This flexibility allows the designer to accommodate 'widows' and 'orphans' – that is pages that start with the last line of a previous paragraph, or end with a heading, or the first line of a new paragraph. In traditional settings the internal spacing is sometimes stretched or squeezed in order to force the text to finish at the same point on each page. Normally this has little effect in pages of continuous prose, but there are occasions when such a policy can mislead the reader into thinking that they have finished a page when in fact there is more text to follow.

2.2.2 Horizontal spacing

In this textbook all of the lines of text are set 'justified'. This means that they are all equally long and that the text has straight left- and right-hand edges or margins. Such a procedure is common in printed texts. The straight edges are achieved by varying the spacing between the words on each line and, occasionally, by hyphenating or breaking the words at the ends of lines. Indeed, in text with very narrow columns (e.g. in newspapers or some medical leaflets), the spaces between the letters forming the actual words are varied in order to force the text to fit the given line length.

A different approach is to provide a consistent space between each word – producing 'unjustified' text. Here there is the same amount of space between

Writing health communication

each word, and there are usually no word-breaks (or hyphens) at the ends of the lines. Consequently the text has a ragged right-hand edge. Most screen-based text is like this, and it is becoming common practice in more informal health-related medical communications (such as patient information leaflets).

There has been much debate over the relative merits of justified and unjusti-fied printed text. It would appear that it does not matter much which setting is used as far as understanding conventional text is concerned: the decision con-cerning which format to use is largely one of choice. There is some evidence, however, that unjustified text might be more helpful for less able readers, whether they are younger children or older adults (see Hartley, 2004a).

Unjustified text has other advantages. For example, we can – if we wish – specify that no line should end with the first word of a new sentence or that, if the last word on a line is preceded by a punctuation mark, then this last word should be carried over to start the next line. And, of course, it is possible to con-sider the starting points of each line too. Indentation can be used to convey sub-structure (as shown in Figure 2.3).

For adults and children over 12

   Take 1 or 2 tablets with food 2 or 3 times a day.

   Do not take more than 6 tablets in 24 hours.

   Leave at least 4 hours between doses.

Do not give this medicine to children under 12.

Do not take this medicine during pregnancy.

   It may delay labour or

   make it last longer.

Figure 2.3   Revised spatial arrangement of the text shown in Figure 2.2

2.2.3 Combining vertical and horizontal spacing

For all texts, inter-related decisions have to be taken that depend upon the nature of the text. If, for example, the text consists of continuous prose, then (on a smallish page) a single-column structure with normal paragraph indentation may be perfectly acceptable. If, however, the text consists of numerous small ele-ments, many of which start on new lines, then using traditional indentation to denote new paragraphs will be misleading. It is for reasons such as these that I generally advocate the use of line-spacing rather than indentation to denote the start of new paragraphs in instructional and informational text (see Hartley, 2004a). Figure 2.3 above shows the same text as that shown in Figure 2.2 but now both the vertical and the horizontal spacing of the text have been manipu-lated to clarify its meaning.

Designing easy-to-read text

In Figure 2.4, the same text has been parsed by computer, using one of the programs developed by Walker et al. (2007). Such computer programs analyse the natural language content of the text – primarily syntactic structures, but also word difficulty and patterns of punctuation – and then specify formatting patterns (e. g., line breaks and indentations) to optimise the perception and the linguistic processing of the content. Research shows that readers recall more from text set in this manner compared to traditional settings (Walker et al., 2007). Furthermore, when people are asked to recall short texts set in these different formats, they usually write them out in the ways that they were presented (Hartley, 1993).

```
For adults and children
    over 12,
    take 1 or 2 tablets
        with food,
    2 or 3
        times a day.

Do not take
    more than 6 tablets
    in 24 hours.

Leave at least 4 hours
    between doses.

Do not give
    this medicine
        to children under 12.

Do not take this medicine
    during pregnancy.

It may delay labour,
    or make it last longer.
```

Figure 2.4   Revised spatial arrangement of the text shown in Figure 2.2 with spacing determined by computer (see Walker et al., 2007). Figure courtesy of Randall Walker

2.2.4 Big mistakes

The US presidential election in 2000 provided an example of the difficulties that can arise when the spacing of the text is not properly considered. Here many voters in Florida found themselves voting inadvertently for the arch Republican (Pat Buchanan) rather than the Democratic candidate (Al Gore) because the punch-holes for voting for each candidate were not systematically aligned to the candidates' names (see illustration in Hartley, 2004b). As it happened, because Florida was a key state in the election, many Florida voters became unintentionally instrumental in the election of George Bush to the presidency.

This is an extreme example, but text should *not* be designed, as so often happens, on a 'Let's put this here' basis. Decisions concerning the vertical and the horizontal spacing of the text need to be made in advance of setting it, and these decisions need to be kept throughout the text. When a text contains a mixture of text, diagrams, and other instructional materials, then the writers and designers have to think much harder about the best ways of presenting the materials and how to do it systematically. In particular, things to avoid are placing such different elements at random on the page, and printing over or round photographs and illustrations.

Designers typically use what is called a 'typographical reference grid' to achieve a uniform rather than a messy approach (e.g., see Hartley, 2004a; Tondreau, 2009). This tool – which allows layout decisions to be mapped out in advance on a hidden underlay or grid – allows the designer to plan for standard units of space to separate out each of the components within the text. Thus, for example, one can specify in advance the width of the outer and inner margins and the text, the normal and the maximum number of lines per page, and how many units of linespace to allow between the text and tables or figures and their captions, and so on.

2.3 Choosing type-sizes and typefaces

2.3.1 Type-sizes

Many researchers have suggested appropriate type-sizes for reading and give advice on related issues such as line-length and line-spacing. Tinker (1963) provides good summaries of the earlier literature in this respect, and Schriver (1997) provides a more up to date account.

Unfortunately, much of the early research on type-sizes is not very helpful for the designers of health-related texts. This is principally because the variables such as type-size, line-length and interline-spacing were not studied in the 'real-life' context of such materials. Most early researchers, for example, considered issues of type-size with very short, simple settings of continuous prose or meaningless text (e.g. see examples in Hartley, 2004a).

Today there are many different measurement systems used in the printing industry but, with the advent of electronic printing, one might imagine, perhaps naively, that these will be rationalised. One particular measure that has remained for some reason is that of the 'point'. (Somewhat oversimplifying it, a point measures 0.0138 inches or 0.3527 mm.) Typical type-sizes in textbooks and on screen are 10, 11 and 12 point. The 'small print' (in legal documents, for example) may be 6 or 8 point, but this is too small for most people to read with ease. Larger sizes (such as 14, 18 and 24 point) are normally used for headings and display. The typographic setting of a text is often described, for example, as '10 on 12' point. This indicates that there is an extra space of two points between the lines of print to facilitate reading.

Another confusing aspect of this research is that people recommend specific type-sizes without regard for the fact that the size of a particular typeface (say, 12 point) does *not* refer to the size of the image as seen by the reader. The specified size refers only to the depth of space required (originally) by a line of metal type when it was set with minimum line-to-line spacing. However, letters also vary in terms of their horizontal widths.

Figure 2.5, for instance, shows text printed in one size of type but in five different typefaces. As can be seen, the width of the letters varies even when the vertical dimension is constant.

For adults and children over 12 (Times New Roman)

For adults and children over 12 (Palatino)

For adults and children over 12 (Century Gothic)

For adults and children over 12 (Bookman Old Style)

For adults and children over 12 (Courier New)

Figure 2.5   Text set in different 12-point typefaces

Clearly no single typeface or type style can be recommended. Designers need to examine their texts carefully to avoid problems that can arise if they choose too small or too large a typeface and too long or short a particular line-length. For example, it is probably easier to read:

> Leaving the leather strap in damp areas can cause it to go mouldy or to crack. To ensure a long life for the band ...

than:

> Leaving the leather strap in damp areas
> can cause it to go mouldy or to crack. To
> ensure a long life for the band ...

Health-related materials, including patient information leaflets, have to be read close-up, and most manufacturers print them in tiny type-sizes, thus making them unreadable. As a rule of thumb, text set in 12 point type with one-and-a-half line-spacing can be read by most people (including those with minor visual impairments).

So designers need to examine their texts carefully to avoid problems that can arise if they choose *too small* or *too large* a typeface. For example, in posters, the use of large type-sizes means that each line will only contain three or four words at most. In this case it is difficult to group the words syntactically in each line. Small type-sizes will allow you to include a good deal of information on each line – but at what cost if the text is unreadable?

Writing health communication

2.3.2 Typefaces

Today there are today several thousands, if not millions, of typefaces available. So how does one decide which one(s) to use? In practice, as Black (1990) pointed out, choosing a typeface really means:

1 Considering the purpose of the text.
2 Making sure that the chosen sizes and weights required for the text (e.g. light, medium, bold) are available.
3 Making sure that the character set contains not only the commonly used signs but also any additional special characters called for by the text (e.g., mathematical symbols).
4 Considering how well particular typefaces will withstand repeated copying.

Certain typefaces seem more appropriate in some situations than others. Neither 'jokerman', for example, nor '**Impact**' would seem useful for health-related text, although they may be appropriate for party invitations. Some readers have personal preferences for particular typefaces, and others have pointed out that some typefaces have emotional connotations. These individual differences suggest that it is wiser to keep to conventional and familiar typefaces than it is to use idiosyncratic ones.

2.3.3 Serifs and sans-serifs

Typefaces are typically classified into those that have serifs (finishing strokes at the ends of letters) and those that do not (sans-serifs). For example, in Figure 2.5 above, the top example is printed in a serif typeface (Times New Roman) and the third a sans-serif typeface (Century Gothic).

Unfortunately, research gives no clear guidance about which style is best either for printed or electronic text. Some designers of printed texts recommend that faces with serifs be used for the body of the text and that faces without serifs be used for headings, or for other purposes (such as to differentiate the examples from the body of the text). Others consider that typefaces without serifs are more legible in the smaller sizes (e.g. 8 and 10 point) and go on to argue that such sans-serif typefaces are better for text that is not intended for continuous reading (e.g. reference works, tables, catalogues, etc.). Others indeed suggest that sans-serif faces might be more appropriate for older readers.

Schriver (1997) reviews much of the relevant literature here for printed text. She concludes that one has to make decisions that are based upon good practice and common sense. I would add, too, that there are so many different typefaces *within* each of the major groupings (serif or sans-serif) that it makes little sense to generalise in terms of comparing faces with serifs with those without them. It is better to consider how different particular typefaces compare in the context of the planned text.

Dyson (2005) makes similar comments when examining research on screen-based typefaces. Here there is little actual research but what there is supports the

Designing easy-to-read text

use of sans-serif faces. Bernard and Mills (2000), for instance, recommended using 12 point Arial rather than 12 point Times Roman in a study with adults, and Bernard, Chaparro, Mills and Halcomb (2002) made similar recommendations from a study with children. Ling and van Schaik (2006) found no significant differences in information retrieval from screen-based text set in 12-point Times Roman and 10-point Arial, but they recommended, on the basis of their users' preferences, using sans-serif Arial. Mackiewicz (2007) similarly found few differences between judgments of the effectiveness of PowerPoint slides printed in five serif and five sans-serif typefaces, but found that the sans-serif faces were deemed more professional.

2.3.4 Capital letters

PARAGRAPHS OF TEXT SET IN CAPITAL LETTERS ARE MORE DIFFICULT TO READ THAN ARE PARAGRAPHS SET IN UPPER- AND LOWER-CASE LETTERS. THE USE OF STRINGS OF WORDS IN CAPITALS FOR MAIN HEADINGS (OR SMALL CAPITALS FOR SECONDARY HEADINGS) MAY CAUSE FEW PROBLEMS BECAUSE SUCH HEADINGS ARE NORMALLY SURROUNDED BY SPACE THAT AIDS THEIR PERCEPTION. ON THE WHOLE, THOUGH, THE USE OF CAPITAL LETTERS SHOULD BE KEPT TO A MINIMUM. APART FROM THEIR SPECIALISED USE IN MATHEMATICAL WORK, CAPITAL LETTERS ARE BEST RESERVED FOR THE FIRST LETTER OF A SENTENCE (INCLUDING HEADINGS), AND FOR THE FIRST LETTER OF PROPER NOUNS. NOTICES PRINTED IN CAPITAL LETTERS ARE HARD TO READ.

2.3.5 Italics

Sloping or 'italic' characters were originally introduced into printed books in the sixteenth century. With italics you could have more characters to the line, the style of letters being more compressed than the vertically drawn and rounded forms of the normal lower-case character set. It is commonly accepted that continuous italic text is harder to read than the more conventional typographic settings (see Schriver, 1997). Italic is thus more commonly used for signalling other features, such as distinct or especially important words or points.

2.3.6 Bold

Bold text is also often used for emphasis but, like capitals and italic, this should be done sparingly. Bold text loses its effect when there is too much of it.

2.3.7 Numbers and 'bullets'

Numbers or 'bullets' are useful for making a series of points within a paragraph. Compare: 'Four devices to help the reader are a detailed contents page,

Writing health communication

skeleton outlines for each chapter, headings in the text, and a concluding summary...' with:

'Four devices to help the reader are:

1   a detailed contents page,
2   skeleton outlines for each chapter,
3   headings in the text, and
4   a concluding summary.'

It also helps the reader if you use space to list the points in a structurally similar way, e.g.:

Bullet-points for items without any particular order	Numbers for steps in a sequence	Letters for mutually exclusive items
• --------	1 -------	(a) --------
• --------	2 -------	(b) --------
• --------	3 -------	(c) -------

2.3.8 Colour

Colour can be used in medical texts in many different ways. Sometimes, for example, coloured headings may be used simply to make the text more appealing. In other situations subordinate text may be set in a different colour in order to differentiate it from the main content.

There is a considerable amount of research on the effectiveness of colour cueing in printed instructional texts and multi-media presentations. As it happens, there appear to be few clear generalisations that one can make but it is important to remember that:

* readers have colour preferences;
* readers like some additional colour;
* colour can help learning; but
* extra colours have to be used sparingly and consistently, if they are not to confuse the readers;
* some colours stand out more than others, so it is unhelpful to use a range of colours on the same page or screen;
* certain combinations of colours are more legible than others in print or on screen. Thus, for example, black ink on white or yellow paper is generally preferable to red ink on these colours, and black ink on dark red or purple background is generally to be avoided.
* certain colours and combinations of colours do not copy well in black and white, so the details may get lost when black and white copies are made.

Designing easy-to-read text

- about 8.5 per cent of males and 0.5 per cent of females are colour blind, to some extent;
- there is considerable debate about the value of different coloured papers, screens (and overlays) for dyslexic readers (Wilkins, 2003).

2.3.9 Combining typographic cues

All of these devices for emphasising different aspects of the text need to be used sparingly for they lose their significance if they are used in combination or excessively. Nor is it wise to present readers with text that continually changes in size, in spacing and in typeface. A brief rule of thumb is that there is no need to use three or more additional cues to emphasise something when one or two at most will do.

2.4 Size matters

IMPORTANT NOTICE
IT IS OUR PRACTICE POLICY
THAT ANY TREATMENT CARRIED OUT ON YOUR
APPOINTMENT HAS TO BE PAID FOR THIS DAY

Notices such as the one above have to be read at a distance, and most people print them in larger letters than normal. Some use capitals letters, some bold, some colour, and some underline. Some do all four which is confusing. As a rule of thumb, larger lower-case letters set in 24-point type in black can be read at a distance of 3 feet or 1 metre. A better design for the notice above might be:

Important notice

Any treatment carried out on the day of your appointment has to be paid for that day.

2.5 Conclusions

To conclude, I provide a list of do's and don'ts. I suggest that guides such as the ones discussed above should be thought about carefully, rather than slavishly followed. And, in all cases, the resulting text needs to be tested with samples of appropriate readers before being finalised.

Do:

- Consider the purpose of the text, and how best to achieve these aims.
- Choose an appropriate page size.
- Plan the page arrangements in advance, especially if there are illustrative materials to be included.
- Decide in advance on the amount of space to be used to separate each of the sub-components of the text (e.g., headings, paragraphs, illustrations, captions).
- Think about using a line-space rather than indentation to separate the paragraphs.
- Consider using unjustified text.
- Try the text out with a mixture of appropriate readers.

Do not:

- Use inappropriate type-sizes (and typefaces).
- Over-use the numbers of cues available for emphasising text (especially capital letters, underlining and colour).
- Use a 'Let's put this here' approach to deciding where to place tables, graphs, and illustrations, etc.

Good luck!

References

Bernard, M.L., Chaparro, B.S., Mills, M.M. and Halcomb, C. (2002) 'Examining children's reading performance and preference for different computer-displayed text', *Behaviour & Information Technology*, 21(2): 87–96.

Bernard, M.L. and Mills, M.M. (2000) 'So, what size and type of font should I use on my website?' *Usability News*, 2(2): 1–5.

Black, A. (1990) *Typefaces for Desktop Publishing: A User Guide*. London: Architecture Design and Technology Press.

Dyson, M.C. (2005) 'How do we read texts on screen?' In H. van Oostendorp, L. Breure and A. Dillon (eds), *Creation, Use, and Deployment of Digital Information*. Mahwah, NJ: Erlbaum, pp. 279–306.

Fisher, D. (1976) 'Spatial factors in reading and research: the case for space', in R. A. Monty and J. W. Senders (eds), *Eye-Movements and Psychological Processes*. Hillsdale, NJ: Erlbaum, pp. 417–28.

Hartley, J. (1993) 'Recalling structured text: does what goes in determine what comes out?' *British Journal of Educational Technology*, 24(3): 85–91.

Hartley, J. (2004a) 'Designing instructional and informational text', in D. H. Jonassen (ed.), *Handbook of Research in Educational Communications and Technology* (2nd edn). Mahwah, NJ: Erlbaum.

Designing easy-to-read text

Hartley, J. (2004b) 'Applying psychology to text design: a personal view', *Information Design Journal and Document Design*, 12(2): 91–102.

Hartley, J. and Johnson, M. (2000) 'Portrait or landscape? Typographical layouts for patient information leaflets', *Visible Language*, 34(3): 296–309.

Ling, J. and van Schaik, P. (2006) 'The influence of font type and line length on visual search and information retrieval in web pages', *International Journal of Human-Computer Studies*, 64(5): 395–404.

Ling, J. and van Schaik, P. (2007) 'The influence of line spacing and text alignment on visual search of web pages', *Displays*, 28(2): 60–7.

Mackiewicz, J. (2007) 'Audience perceptions of fonts in projected PowerPoint slides', *Technical Communication*, 54(3): 295–307.

Schriver, K.A. (1997) *Dynamics of Document Design*. New York: Wiley.

Small, J.P. (1997) *Wax Tablets of the Mind: Cognitive Studies of Classical Antiquity*. New York: Routledge.

Tinker, M.A. (1963) *Legibility of Print*. Ames: Iowa State University Press.

Tondreau, B. (2009) *Layout Essentials: 100 Design Principles for Using Grids*. Massachusetts: Rockport Publishers Inc.

Walker, R.C., Schloss, P., Gordon, A.S., Vogel, C.A., Fletcher, R. and Walker, S.D. (2007) 'Visual-syntactic-text-formatting: theoretical basis and empirical evidence for impact on human reading', in *Proceedings of the Institute for Electronic Engineers (IEEE) International Professional Communication Conference (IPCC) of the Professional Communications Society (PCS)*, 'Engineering the Future of Human Communication', Seattle, 1–3 October.

Wilkins, A. (2003) *Reading Through Colour: How Coloured Filters Can Reduce Reading Difficulty, Eyes Strain and Headaches*. London: Wiley.

3

Making written materials easy to understand

Marieke Kools

Helping people change their behaviour is a primary aim of health promotion. In order to change their behaviour, people need to understand *why* they should change and *how* they can change. Changes range from establishing long-term physical activity patterns to improved use of medication or aids. Brochures and leaflets are often used to motivate readers. Understanding the message is essential in facilitating behavioural change and in this chapter we focus on enhancing understanding of written text.

Learning Outcomes

After reading this chapter, you should be able to:

1 Analyse texts for clarity and identify strong and weak points.
2 Choose among several techniques to repair textual incoherence and enhance clarity for your target audience.
3 Judge what kind of graphic support may help readers understand the message.
4 Develop a critical and constructive perspective on improving graphical aids in your own written materials.
5 Design effective graphical aids such as graphic organisers, pictorials and icons, and illustrations.
6 Test the comprehensibility of your materials and identify potential improvements.

Information processing theories clarify that comprehension is critical to acceptance and persuasiveness of messages (McGuire, 1972). To help readers understand, accept and act on written messages, textual and graphic features should facilitate understanding. Of course, all health promoters are aware of this. Nowadays, almost all brochures and leaflets make use of headings, pictures and diagrams. However, given the power of graphics to communicate in a glance, the way in which graphics are used is critical. This chapter will provide examples of good and bad graphic design, explaining each case. We begin with a brief sketch of how readers interpret text and graphics.

3.1 Cognitive mechanisms underlying comprehension

Figure 3.1 shows an overview of the mental processes that take place when readers read a text or interpret a graph. Please examine the diagram closely.

When reading a text (see Figure 3.1: step 1) its contents are processed in the reader's working memory (WM) by representing or encoding concepts as they are sequentially encountered (see step 2). These concepts can be new to the reader or familiar, indicated by the two paths that lead to 'integration in WM'. Readers form a mental representation of what they read by continually connecting incoming text information (step 3) with existing knowledge stored in their long-term memory (LTM) (step 4). Comprehension of the information in the text takes place when the reader can identify each new piece of text information and relate it to the information already given. Bearing this in mind, the following two guidelines are vital for effective text design:

1   Only a limited number of concepts can be held active in working memory at any point in time. Therefore, it is important that not too many concepts are introduced in a particular section of text and that those concepts are repeated.
2   Graphic and textual elements should match perfectly and leave no room for ambiguity.

Considering these statements, and Figure 3.1, some features of good and bad design become evident. You may have found yourself rereading some pieces of text, asking yourself questions like 'Why is that box included?', 'Where is the text explaining that element of Figure 3.1?'. You may have wondered where it is that step five in the figure is explained (you are correct, it is not yet). Maybe you even were getting a bit irritated, thinking that this is not a clear illustration – especially for a chapter discussing how to use graphics. This is typically how readers respond to difficult text and unclear graphics.

Figure 3.1 has strengths and weaknesses. It is a good diagram because it provides a concise overview of crucial elements, which are explained textually. In the text, each step explicitly refers to specific elements in the figure, to enable mental connections between important elements and so enhance understanding of the process explained. What may have confused you when 'reading' this diagram, is that several graphic and textual elements were not explained before you looked at the figure and you may have found yourself guessing at the meaning. This is rather obvious bad design but it is not that uncommon in existing health promotion materials. We will consider both textual and graphic elements that have been found to aid the mental connection process underpinning comprehension of readers and we will try to improve the clarity of Figure 3.1

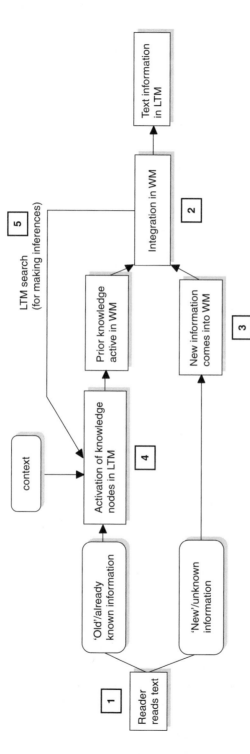

Figure 3.1 Overview of the mental processes that take place when readers read a text or interpret a graph (see Kools et al., 2004)

Note: LTM: Long term memory   WM: Working memory

3.2 Constructing text that is easy to understand

Readers are not aware of textual coherence when text is well constructed but a lack of coherence attracts (negative) attention. Readers' prior knowledge is critical. The more that the textual information coincides with what readers already know, the easier it will be for them to integrate 'new' information into their existing 'knowledge base', hence coming to understand the material presented. As is shown in Figure 3.1 (element 5), when 'new' and 'old/known' information do not coincide, readers make 'inferences' to establish comprehension. McNamara and colleagues (McNamara et al., 1996) showed that this 'mental work', also called 'active processing', is necessary for comprehension to occur. They found, counter-intuitively, that when readers with ample prior knowledge read a very coherent text, they remembered less than similarly knowledgeable readers who read a less coherent text. The inferences which the latter group had to make led to more 'active processing' of the text and helped them to understand the information. Of course, readers must be able to make the necessary inferences, otherwise the comprehension process breaks down. However, the key point is that by prompting inferences which the reader can easily make, we enhance comprehension by actively engaging the reader. Thus, we come to another major point for designers to keep in mind:

> health promotion materials designers should know what kind of experiences and knowledge their audience is likely to have in order to calculate what textual elements can be omitted or left implicit for readers to infer or 'mentally connect' for themselves

Having established who the members of your target audience are and what they know, you may then choose what to explain and how. The '*what*' being a matter of content, is covered in Chapters 6–10. In this chapter we focus on the '*how*'. Text is clearer, when the principles of prior knowledge and inference are applied to sentences and links between sentences as well as to graphics and their explanations. The last sentence that is read provides the prior knowledge required to interpret the sentence that follows. When sentences are effectively linked with each other, a text is said to be *coherent*. Several principles to make texts coherent have been established in the field of cognitive psychology. These are explained below.

3.2.1 Writing text: macro and micro elements

A text has two different levels at which it can be coherent: the global and the local level, also called the macro level and micro level, respectively. At both levels, readers need to maintain coherence in their mental representation of a text to understand its content (Lorch et al., 1985). A text is coherent at the macro level when the order of topics is logical as opposed to random and if the text sections are clearly related to each other and to the overall topic. For example, your readers may generally expect to read about causes, effects and 'things to do about those causes'. Starting with the 'things to do' makes little sense if readers have not yet read the reasons justifying the actions you describe. Thus, starting with reasons and then providing instructions makes a text more coherent at the macro level.

At the micro level, a text is coherent if each sentence is explicitly related to the next. Consequently, readers do not have to infer relationships between sections and sentences by themselves. This is (quite logically) called 'inference reduction': the links between concepts are there, made explicit in the text. For example, by repeating the subject of the previous sentence in the sentence that follows, there is no doubt that the second sentence still refers to the same thing. When a pronoun or synonym is used instead of that same subject-word, readers need to be able to 'mentally replace' that pronoun with the subject-word from the previous sentence. This can create room for error. And knowing Murphy's Law, it may be better to be safe than sorry. At both the macro and micro level, coherence can be increased by applying specific writing principles to the text. These principles are outlined in the set of guidelines below.

3.2.2 Core text design guidelines

For textual coherence at the macro level, in an iterative writing process, i.e., a writing process in which one goes through the same cycles several times, writers and editors should ensure that their texts comprise the following two features:

1 headings are used to flag content.
2 The first and last sentences in paragraphs should explain how the information relates to previous and upcoming information, respectively.

For textual coherence on the text's micro level, seven principles should be kept in mind while (re)writing a text:

1 Repeat the linking word from the previous sentence to maintain argument overlap.
2 Only use demonstrative pronouns (this, that, these, those) when they have only one possible referent to avoid ambiguity.
3 Add descriptive elaborations to explain difficult or unusual words.
4 Use sentence connectives to clarify relationships between sentences.
5 Maintain a 'given-new' order of information within sentences.
6 Explicitly state the actor in each sentence.
7 Pay special attention to explicating causality, possibly by using these principles.

3.2.3 Additional text design guidelines

Research has also highlighted a series of additional principles consistent with psychological understanding of text (Davis et al., 1998; Doak et al., 1996). These also follow from a cognitive perspective on text processing and comprehension. Thus, the following principles are useful additions to those listed above:

1 Sentences should not be too long; i.e., no more than one new concept should be introduced in a sentence.

Making written materials easy to understand

2 Use the active voice instead of the passive voice.
3 The main verb should be at the beginning of the sentence, rather than the end.
4 Add concrete, highly imaginable examples when possible.
5 Delete irrelevant or distracting information.

We conducted a study into the use of these guidelines by Dutch health education text writers and found great diversity in their use of these principles (Kools et al., 2004). An explicit awareness of these principles when writing and editing text may ensure more consistent application which, in turn, may lead to more coherent and more easily understood health promotion texts. In addition, use of these principles when pre-testing materials prior to publication, may identify and facilitate repair to comprehension breakdowns – which brings us to the matter of testing for comprehensibility.

3.2.4 Testing for textual coherence

The principles above provide you with tools for a critical analysis of your own text in which you can examine each pronoun, each long sentence and each explanation. However, as a health promotion specialist, the knowledge you have is much more extensive than that of your target readers. No matter how well you feel you can identify and empathise with their experience and understand what they know and which inferences they will be able to make, you can never be sure until you test your text with target readers. The most valuable information is gained by having a reader from your target audience read your text and mark wherever they are unsure of, have to re-read (parts of) a sentence or do not understand. Even without any further interview or discussion with the reader, you may be able to improve the text considerably, just by applying the principles above to each point marked. Feedback from only a few, say three people, could allow you to improve as much as 80 per cent of potentially 'difficult' text.

If you have doubts about a piece of text, or if it is very important that a particular section of the text is properly understand, you may want to ask test readers some questions about that section. Asking a test reader whether they did or did not understood (so they can answer 'yes' or 'no') may lead the reader to dismiss doubts and raise concerns about whether their doubts are due to their own intellect rather than shortcomings in the text. Therefore, it is important to do the following:

Test your materials in the most objective way as possible.

You can do this by asking content-related questions, such as: 'What was the main point made in this paragraph?', 'Please explain in your own words what was said/ how X works.' Be specific in your questions and do not provide multiple choices for answers. The kinds of answers readers give to these open-ended questions can provide valuable insights into what exactly they misunderstood, or did not remember, or even disagreed with. We will say more about pre-testing later in this chapter and in subsequent chapters.

Writing health communication

3.3 Understanding graphics

Graphics may be used for several purposes in health promotion materials. They may help to attract readers' attention, locate answers, explain, give instructions, or support numerical understanding. In this section we would like to elaborate further on the two purposes of graphics, which are both comprehension-related, namely the purposes of 'explaining', and 'giving instructions'. Interestingly, although some graphic elements may be designed primarily to enhance comprehension, they may also serve additional purposes, intended or otherwise. One particular type of graphic, a graphic organiser, may provide insight into a leaflet's macro-structure, thus enhancing comprehension of the main points. A graphic organiser can also clarify the information sequence and therefore help readers to locate information in the text. In addition, icons or pictorials that help understand the type of information they refer to may make the materials more attractive and thus invite readers to read through them. The examples below illustrate these points and show you how different graphics can be used.

3.3.1 Graphic organisers

Graphic organisers depict relationships among concepts in the text. They are known aids for text comprehension in the area of instructional design (Dee-Lucas and Larkin, 1995) but are not widely known among health promotion specialists. Graphic organisers are based on purely textual 'advance organisers'. An advance organiser is a simple, short piece of text explaining what follows, by using for example, a metaphor, to help the reader grasp relatively technical textual explanation or instructions. The goal of the advance organiser is to make the interpretation and thus understanding of the difficult information easier, because readers can follow a familiar line of thought which was presented immediately before (hence the term 'advance organiser'). For example, to explain the difficult concept of gravitational pull between planets, an advance organiser explaining what happens if you tie two balls to each other with a rope and swing one ball around, could help readers grasp the concept more easily. A 'graphic organiser' has the same purpose – to provide a basic plan or way of thinking about upcoming, more difficult information. The only difference is, that it is a *graphic* depiction instead of a purely textual one. We use the words 'graphic organiser' to refer only to diagrams but other writers include illustrations or photographs in their definition. Figure 3.2 shows some examples of what we mean by 'graphic organisers'.

Looking at the four organisers shown, your next question may be: How can I design an effective graphic organiser? Many design choices can be made and the right choice depends very much on *what* you want to introduce or explain with your organiser.

Research into how people represent their knowledge mentally, has shown that they do this in a hierarchical way. The defining feature of a hierarchy is that it represents multiple 'levels' of concepts with the main purpose of communicating superordinate–subordinate concept relationships. This may account for findings that hierarchical overviews, for instance in the form of tree diagrams, facilitate

Making written materials easy to understand

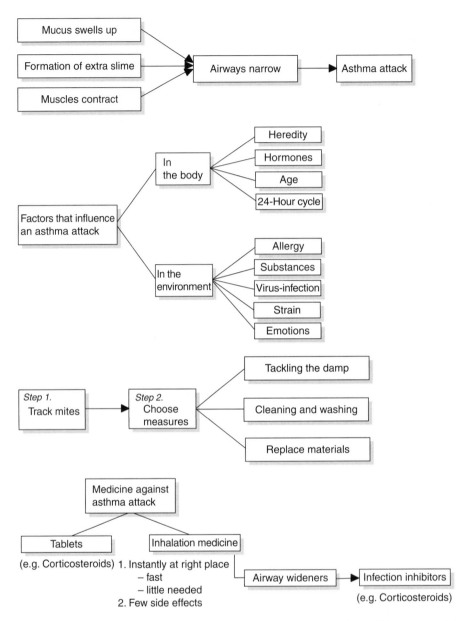

Figure 3.2 Translated examples (originally in Dutch) of the four different graphic organisers used to represent each main subject in a leaflet about asthma. Note that arrows indicate some temporal sequence, whereas for mere linkage of concepts, normal lines are used. Each figure was presented at the top of the page above the text it referred to

comprehension of the thematic structure of a text because they make it easier for readers to organise information in memory (Lorch et al., 1993). Tree diagrams have consistently been found to be most effective for learning when compared to plain texts and network maps.

We devised multiple graphic organisers in line with the findings explained above to aid comprehension of an extensive, mostly textual leaflet for parents of children with asthma (Kools et al., 2006a). Specifically, the four graphic organisers shown in Figure 3.2 were developed, corresponding with the four main themes of the brochure text. The organisers presented the same information and relationships among concepts as were outlined in the text. They were hierarchical in nature, in the sense that concepts were interconnected from left to right to communicate superordinate–subordinate relationships (Wallace et al., 1998). Apart from the first page, a graphic organiser was placed at the top of all the pages. Relevant concepts on each particular page were highlighted in the organiser by means of thick lines and shadings. Thus, in addition to showing and highlighting relationships between important concepts in the text, the organisers also served to identify content and so could assist readers in finding information.

We found that readers' text comprehension improved when they read the brochure with the four graphic organisers. Improvements in textual understanding were found in relation to both micro- and macro- level concepts. Not only were participants better able to recall global and specific information more easily, they also showed superior performance when explaining processes and applying this knowledge to different situations. Thus, the graphic organisers helped the readers not only to grasp the macro structure of the text but also facilitated memory and comprehension of detailed, micro-level text information. It seems likely that the graphic organisers provided a ready-made structure which helped readers organise what they had learnt in their memory.

Finally, some graphic organiser guidelines:

1   When readers need to understand and use the knowledge acquired from a health education text, health promotion specialists may consider explaining relationships between concepts in the text using graphic organisers.
2   Graphic organisers should show the hierarchical relationships between concepts. Temporal and causal relationships may be represented with arrows from causes to effects.
3   The diagrams used in graphic organisers should not be too extensive, that is, not have more than three levels and preferably only two.
4   The organiser should be placed in close proximity to the text that it represents, because otherwise readers may miss the relationship between the visual and textual information.
5   If a graphic organiser covers text on several pages it should appear at the top of every page with relevant concepts on that page highlighted in the organiser with thicker lines and shadings.

3.3.2 Illustrations

In the previous section we showed you that when explaining something in a text, a clarifying visual aid may help. In addition to graphic organisers, simple line-drawings can help the reader visualise what otherwise would be left to their own

Making written materials easy to understand

sometimes unpredictable imaginations. We know from instructional design research that the presence of pictorial information allows readers to visualise relations in the text, which may enhance comprehension of its contents. In a similar fashion as was explained in the model depicted in Figure 3.1, visual representations are mentally linked with textual representations in working memory. Readers are better able to build connections between these two types of representations when the corresponding text and picture are held in working memory at the same time (Baddeley, 1986). Working memory is limited in time and processing capacity, so this concurrent activation is most likely to happen when text and illustrations are presented together, illustrating a 'spatial-contiguity effect' (Moreno and Mayer, 1999). One probably familiar design guideline emanating from these insights, is the use of 'captions'. Adding textual captions to illustrations to explain important aspects of the picture's content can help this simultaneous processing in working memory.

When considering the use of illustrations to promote comprehension it may be useful to think about the following issues.

First, it is important to know *what kind of information* it is that one wants to clarify. Different kinds of text may be supported by adding illustrations. For example, explanations of technical or temporal processes may especially benefit from appropriate illustrations. You may think of explanations of bodily functions, the process of becoming ill, or the intake and workings of medication. When describing an unchanged or static state of affairs, one simple line-drawing may suffice. However, if consecutive steps need to be taken or processes need to be understood, a sequence of illustrations may be necessary to fully cover the text content and prevent readers from mixing up the temporal sequence they need to understand.

Second, the added-value of illustrations can be assessed by considering how self-evident the text describing a situation, a device or process is. The less concrete or imaginable the target information is, the greater the potential added value of an illustration. Unless your readers are doctors or medical specialists themselves, processes in the body typically are unfamiliar and thus difficult to understand. Visualising such non-concrete elements always helps comprehension. With technical, product- or procedural information, the added value of illustrations may vary.

In cognitive ergonomics, a research area devoted to understanding and improving the usability of information, such inherent clarity is described in terms of 'affordances' and 'constraints' (Norman, 1988). Affordances refer to characteristics of objects that are perceived by their users regarding their potential use: objects permit and even provoke certain user-actions because of their form, weight or materials. For instance, a smooth round red button lifted a centimetre from a surface, affords pushing it. Constraints, on the other hand, refer to an object's characteristics that limit possible actions. Scissors, for instance, have two holes with different sizes, limiting the number of fingers you can put through each of them, and the scissors only move in one direction. These constraints help the user identify the scissors' proper use. Thus, the function of a device may be inherently clear, or require minimal explanation. Visual information may add very little in such circumstances. To illustrate both the presence and lack of inherent clarity in design, Figure 3.3 shows two examples of illustration sequences of two medical devices for people with asthma, which vary in their inherent clarity: an inhaler chamber and a peak flow meter.

Use of the inhaler chamber

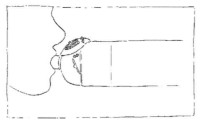

Check whether both valves (ventiles) can move. You can do this by breathing in an out of the inhaler.

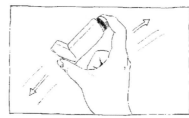

Shake the pump well.

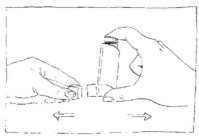

Take the closing cap from the pump.

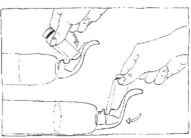

Put the pump into the inhaler chamber.

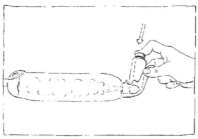

Bring one spray into the inhaler chamber.

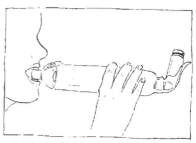

Put the mouthpiece of the inhaler chamber between your teeth. You should close your lips around the mouth piece.

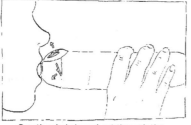

Breath calmly in and out through the inhaler chamber, making the valves move.

Breathing in and out approximately 5-10 times suffices.

Making written materials easy to understand

Use of the peak flow meter.

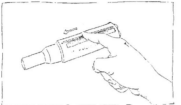

Before blowing, move the indicator back to the bottom of the scale. The indicator is as close to the mouth piece as possible.

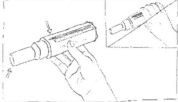

Take care to leave the opening for blowing free and that the indicator can move freely.

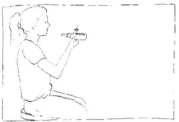

You should take an upright posture e.g. standing or sitting up straight.
When blowing, the scale should be on top.

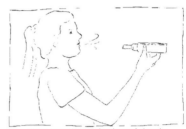

Then breathe in slowly and deeply.

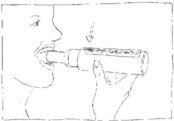

Then put the mouth piece in the mouth, on the tongue; close the teeth and lips around the mouth piece.

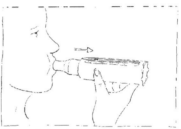

Blow as fast and hard as possible - a short, powerful boost (as if blowing out a candle).

The point of the indicator shows the proper reading.

In total do three attempts according to the method described above. Take a short break (10 seconds) between each attempt and move back the indicator.

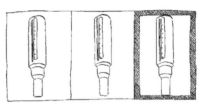

The attempt with the highest value counts. This value is noted (so don't calculate the average value from the three attempts!).

Figure 3.3   Instructions for using an inhaler chamber and a peak flow meter, accompanied by simple illustrations. Notice how the text is in close proximity to the illustrations, making it easy for readers to relate the relevant text to the picture. More space is left vertically between illustrations than horizontally, inviting readers to read the sequence from left to right. Arrows are used to point to small-but-essential details, as well as to indicate movements the reader has to make or can expect the device to make. Also note that in the instructions for the peak flow meter an important mistake that people often make, is shown with a diagonal line across the boxed illustration, which although abstract, is commonly associated with a negative, 'not appropriate or not allowed' message

Writing health communication

As can be seen in the illustrations, the inhaler chamber (or spacer) has a small round extended opening on one side of the tube which affords putting it in one's mouth. A curved holder on the other side of the tube is the only place where the inhaler fits, constraining the placement of the pump on the chamber. However, the inhaler chamber also has valves that the user needs to check which may not be so easy to understand. Use of the chamber also involves a sequence of actions that may not be immediately obvious.

The peak flow meter is a tube with one round pointing opening at the front, which affords putting it into one's mouth. The presence of a scale with a pointer that only moves when blowing into the tube contributes to the affordance of blowing into it. Being a non-transparent object with a closed end constraining the possibility for blowing into the wrong end, it would be a challenge to use it differently. The only information that may not be communicated by the device itself pertains to bodily positions when using it; relatively simple 'actions' that people perform daily to some extent and so may not be entirely unfamiliar.

In the original brochure, both sets of instructions were presented without illustrations. In an experiment, we tested whether the presence of these illustrations would help comprehension (Kools et al., 2006b). Since the text consisted of procedural instructions with a strong temporal sequence that readers should adhere to, both sets of instructions were expected to benefit from illustrations. In addition, based on an analysis of both objects in terms of their inherent clarity, or affordances and constraints as explained above, the inhaler chamber was expected to benefit more from the illustrations than the peak flow meter.

This was tested experimentally, by providing four groups of people with one of the devices and either the text-only or an illustrated version of the instructions. We then asked them to recall the information and subsequently monitored them using the device. It was found that participants who had seen illustrations with the inhaler chamber text recalled more information and more instructional steps. They were also better able to follow the instructions correctly on first use, expressed fewer doubts and finished using the device in a shorter time than the participants with only textual instructions. With the more self-evident peak flow meter, the effects of adding illustrations were weaker but still considerable. The illustrations contributed to a better memory for the sequence of steps and participants felt more confident about their actions while using the device.

Interestingly, the observations of participants using the devices provided us with valuable insights into the kinds of mistakes people make when inferring actions from written text alone. Mistakes were especially noticeable with the inhaler chamber text-only group. The first step in these instructions, which required checking to see if the valves were working correctly, confused the participants who didn't know which valves were meant. As the tube also had two places where it could be opened with two flaps, some started squeezing these. Also, many participants were confused as to where and how to put the pump into the chamber. Participants tried to put it in the mouthpiece, put the wrong end of the pump into the right end of the chamber, even opened the chamber itself and put the whole pump inside. One

Making written materials easy to understand

participant even put the wrong end of the device into her mouth instead of the much smaller mouthpiece. These kinds of mistakes were not made by the participant using the inhaler chamber with the illustrated version of the textual/instructions.

With the peak flow meter, mistakes generally involved careless reading, resulting in some participants neglecting some actions altogether. This skipping of actions ranged from not breathing in deeply before blowing into the device, to not putting their teeth around the mouthpiece or forgetting to move the pointer back to the starting point. Altogether, we think that this makes clear that including illustrations is an effective counter against misunderstanding and incorrect understanding by readers. It seems clear that the original instructions in this asthma brochure had not been pre-tested with novice users; otherwise feedback would have led designers to rethink!

We will return to these issues in Chapter 5 but, for now, the following three guidelines may help:

1   Procedural information that needs to be acted upon should present a combination of illustrations in the form of simple line-drawings and text. Unfamiliar actions that are difficult to visualise need illustrations to help readers understand what to do. In general, comprehension of any complex information can be facilitated by use of line-drawings.
2   A careful analysis of devices or materials being described may help determine which parts of materials most need visual support and/or extended text.
3   Subsequent testing of instructions with novice users by observing their actions is crucial to identify comprehension problems that require design adjustments.

3.3.3 Icons

As also described in Chapter 5, icons may be used to identify or emphasise different kinds of content. Text designers should be cautious when using icons in their materials because they can create more confusion than clarity. The difficulty with icons is that, unlike any other pictorial information, they typically stand alone, *replacing* text. As soon as text is needed to understand them, their purpose is lost. Figure 3.4 shows an icon, used by health promotion specialists in a brochure about healthy dieting.

Figure 3.4   An extensive brochure about healthy dieting contained an icon of an arrow, pointing into a square. This icon was placed regularly in the left margin of the page, next to textual references that guided readers to related sections on other pages of the brochure (see Kools et al., 2007)

Any pictorial (such as an icon) is typically designed to refer to the function, or goal of the object it represents in the context in which it is encountered. For example, a simplified line-drawing of a printer that one can click on in a Word

Writing health communication

processing program refers to the printer's function of printing out a document. A well-designed pictorial can communicate a message at a glance, without any language barriers. Similarly, a poorly designed pictorial may not communicate anything or, worse still, provide the wrong message (Wogalter, 1999).

Thus, research into understanding pictorials has shown that their meanings are not generally self-evident. One reason for this is that many pictorials are not well designed and so fail to convey their intended meaning (Sojourner and Wogalter, 1998). The 'concreteness' of pictorials has been established as an essential feature in their comprehension. 'Concreteness' refers to the extent to which pictorials depict objects, places, or people. Hicks, Bell and Wogalter (2003) showed that it is easier for readers to visualise and understand the pictorial's concept or purpose if the pictorial is concrete. Simple and accurate drawings that are easily recognisable as concrete objects in the real world enable readers to instantly understand that pictorial in its textual context.

With this in mind, have another look at the icon shown in Figure 3.4. It is simple, using only few lines. However, it is unclear what the two horizontal brackets (or square) around it mean: are they just aesthetic, or do they have a function in relation to the arrow? Moreover, there is no 'object in the real world' depicted that the arrow coincides with: arrows themselves are abstract and encountered in various contexts, with various purposes.

We tested comprehension of this icon and found that 65 per cent of the participants did not understand it as an 'indicator of references to other pages with related information', even after seeing it in its context. So after reading the brochure, participants in this study ascribed various, incorrect functions to the arrow icon. These ranged from 'make people turn over to the next page', 'highlight information', 'points towards important information', to 'a kind of bulletpoint'. One person said that she did not even recognise the pictorial as an arrow!

Now look at the icons in Figure 3.5 which were used throughout a leaflet about asthma. What do you think they mean? These two icons were supposed to identify information which was either 'important to understand' (icon on the left) or information which referred to 'actions parents can undertake' (icon on the right). Did you guess this before reading the explanation? Chances are you did not. Moreover, in the brochure, the second icon was accompanied by the words 'what to do'. These words capture the essence of the text they accompanied, are clear and concise and, therefore, provide a more appropriate alternative to the ambiguous icon. In this case, adding visual information did not clarify the text and may have confused readers.

Figure 3.5 Two icons used in the leaflet about asthma

Making written materials easy to understand

When the function is to attract attention, icons may be preferred to text and when it is possible to use an icon depicting a concrete and simple object, this may be very effective. For example, if the icon in Figure 3.6 were used to replace the arrow-icon shown in Figure 3.4 it is likely to be easier to understand. It is a simple drawing of an instantly recognisable commonplace object, namely a signpost. Tests showed that all readers understood the function of this icon (Kools et al., 2007).

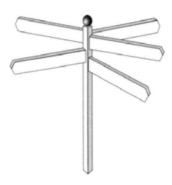

Figure 3.6   An icon of a signpost, as a simple line-drawing, coinciding with a concrete object in the real world, which makes it easy for readers to visualise and thus understand

We should add here that no serious negative consequences are likely to follow from readers' misunderstanding of the icons described above. Most readers probably disregard them altogether or may have been slightly irritated, wondering 'why those are there'. However, incorrectly interpreting icons can have harmful effects. For instance, if icons were used to identify contraindications on a medicine or in a health education brochure and their function was misunderstood, this could have serious consequences (see also Chapter 5). Here are two key guidelines concerning the use of icons in health promotion texts.

1   Only use icons to identify particular kinds of text when concrete, relevant depictions can be designed to accompany the text. If only abstract icons are available and these have no inherent meaning in relation to their function, do not use icons at all. Instead, use brief headings or a single word, possibly in bigger typeface and/or in colour to attract readers' attention.
2   To ensure understanding of an icon's function in context, assess readers' comprehension with open-ended questions. If the information is very important and misunderstanding could lead to harmful outcomes, aim for a minimum of 85 per cent of readers understanding. If the causes of misunderstanding are not potentially harmful, a rate of 67 per cent will suffice.

Writing health communication

3.4 Testing is crucial

Something which all of the studies reported above have in common, is that objective measures were used to test comprehension of materials. Whether or not your text includes graphic organisers, icons, illustrations, or other features, there are ways to test understanding apart from just asking the reader. Asking readers if they understand may not provide an appropriate test because readers may feel obliged to be positive to acknowledge the efforts of the text designers. Also, readers may be hesitant to admit they do not understand or may think they understood something when they did not. This 'illusion of knowing' has been commonly reported in the literature (Glenberg et al., 1982). Using objective measures in which readers are asked to explain the meaning of the text in their own words and, better still, undertake actions described by the text (e.g., using devices) results in more useful insights into what your readers understand. In our study of the graphic organisers, we found exactly that: asking simple questions showed no differences in comprehension between the groups with and without the graphic organisers in the text, whereas using objective measures (of how people used the devices) revealed clear differences in comprehension. We argue that even testing with only a few people from your target audience is worthwhile when objective tests are employed.

3.5 Conclusion

In this chapter we have discussed a number of features that can be included in texts. These include:

1   textual features that prepare readers for demanding text at a global/macro level or the local, micro level of the text;
2   graphic organisers that graphically integrate and summarise the main relationships between relatively abstract concepts outlined in the text;
3   icons that identify or emphasise different kinds of text
4   illustrations that explain textual information visually, by showing the main features and their relationships.

These features may help comprehension of written materials designed to inform readers about their health and take preventive or curative actions. This is their primary aim. Such features may also make the leaflets or brochures more attractive and, thereby, motivate readers to read more carefully. In addition, depending on their use, graphic organisers and icons may make it easier for readers to find specific information they are looking for, thus facilitating accessibility of the materials.

No feature has only one function. Even if it has only one goal in the eyes of the designer, readers may find additional ways to interpret or use a feature.

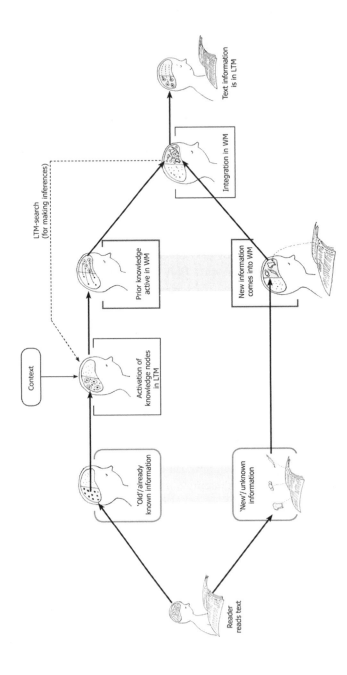

Figure 3.7 Adjusted version of Figure 3.1 (See the colour section at the end of the book) Note how the use of illustrations make the rather abstract psychological explanations easier to envisage and therefore understand and memorise. The colours indicate which elements of the graphics are important and in combination with the slightly differently shaped surrounding lines they link different phases depicted in the graphic₅ with each other

LTM-search
(for making inferences)

Context

Reader
reads text

'Old'/already
known information

'New'/unknown
information

Activation of
knowledge nodes
in LTM

Prior knowledge
active in WM

New information
comes into WM

Integration in WM

Text information
is in LTM

Some design elements, such as the use of colour coding, which are primarily aimed at providing an overview to readers and locating information, may in the end also provide readers with a mental image to categorise and understand different kinds of information. Thus, the design features described in Chapter 4, on the 'usability' of health promotion materials, may also make the information clearer and easier to understand. Designers should be aware of such 'secondary' and unintended effects.

If design features can elicit multiple reactions, *critical evaluation and pre-publication user-testing are essential.* Design features are usually chosen with the best intentions but use of too many or inappropriate features may result in a 'circus' of graphics, reducing readers' ability to locate specific information and understand it. The more concrete and visible you can make a message, the more it is likely to 'stick' for readers. Even after detailed considerations a later revision may allow further improvements. Figure 3.7 is an example of how Figure 3.1, which contained quite technical information, could be further improved. A combination of graphic organiser, illustrations and if possible, the use of colour makes the message clearer and more memorable.

References

Baddeley, A.D. (1986) *Working Memory*. Oxford: Oxford University Press.

Davis, T.C., Michielutte, R., Askov, E.N., Williams, M.V. and Weiss, B.D. (1998) 'Practical assessment of adult literacy in health care', *Health Education and Behavior*, 25, 613–24.

Dee-Lucas, D. and Larkin, J.H. (1995) 'Learning from electronic texts: effects of interactive overviews for information access', *Cognition and Instruction*, 13: 431–68.

Doak, L.G., Doak, C.C. and Meade, C.D. (1996) 'Strategies to improve cancer education materials', *Oncology Nursing Forum*, 23: 1305–12.

Glenberg, A.M., Wilkinson, A.C. and Epstein, W. (1982) 'The illusion of knowing: failure in the self-assessment of comprehension', *Memory and Cognition*, 10: 597–602.

Hicks, K.E., Bell, J.L. and Wogalter, M.S. (2003) 'On the prediction of pictorial comprehension', paper presented at the Human Factors and Ergonomics Society, 47th Annual Meeting, Denver, Colorado.

Kools, M., Ruiter, R.A.C., van de Wiel, M.W.J. and Kok, G. (2004) 'Increasing readers' comprehension of health education brochures: a qualitative study into how professional writers make texts coherent', *Health Education and Behavior*, 31, 720–40.

Kools, M., Van de Wiel, M.W.J., Ruiter, R.A.C., Crüts, A. and Kok, G (2006a) 'The effect of graphic organizers on subjective and objective comprehension of a health education text', *Health Education & Behavior*, 33, 760–72.

Kools, M., Van de Wiel, M.W.J., Ruiter, R.A.C. and Kok, G (2006b) 'Pictures and text in instructions for medical devices: effects on recall and actual performance', *Patient Education & Counseling*, 64, 104–11.

Kools, M., Wright, P., Ruiter, R.A.C., Van de Wiel, M.W.J. and Kok, G. (2007) 'The understandability of pictorials in a health education brochure', internal report, Maastricht University.

Lorch, R.F., Lorch, E.P. and Matthews, P.D. (1985) 'On-line processing of the topic structure of a text', *Journal of Memory and Language*, 24: 350–62.

Lorch, R.F., Lorch, E.P. and Inman, W.E. (1993) 'Effects of signalling topic structure on text recall', *Journal of Educational Psychology*, 85: 281–90.

McGuire, W.J. (1972) 'Attitude change: the information processing paradigm', in C.G. Clintock (ed.), *Experimental Social Psychology*. New York: Holt, Rinehart & Winston.

McNamara, D.S., Kintsch, E., Songer, N.B. and Kintsch, W. (1996) 'Are good texts always better? Interactions of text coherence, background knowledge, and levels of understanding in learning from text', *Cognition and Instruction*, 14: 1–43.

Moreno, R. and Mayer, R.E. (1999) 'Cognitive principles of multimedia learning: the role of modality and contiguity', *Journal of Educational Psychology*, 91: 358–68.

Norman, D. (1988) 'The psychopathology of everyday things', in D. Norman (ed.) *The Psychology of Everyday Things*. New York: Basic Books, pp. 1–33.

Sojourner, R.J. and Wogalter, M.S. (1998) 'The influence of pictorials on the comprehension and recall of pharmaceutical safety and warning information', *International Journal of Cognitive Ergonomics*, 2: 93–106.

Wallace, D.S., West, S.W.C., Ware, A. and Dansereau, D.F. (1998) 'The effect of knowledge maps that incorporate gestalt principles on learning', *The Journal of Experimental Education*, 67: 5–16.

Wogalter, M.S. (1999) 'Factors influencing the effectiveness of warnings', in H.J.G. Zwaga, T. Boersema and H.C.M. Hoonhout (eds), *Visual Information for Everyday Use: Design and Research Perspectives*. London: Taylor & Francis Ltd, pp. 93–110.

4

Making written materials
easy to use

Marieke Kools

Following the previous chapter on how design can aid message comprehension, this chapter will consider the usability of health promotion texts. In the current information-dense society, people have become 'scanners' instead of 'readers' of texts. In practice, health promotion materials are rarely read from start to finish. Instead, people skim through the contents and read whatever catches their interest. And if you are lucky, they will value the contents and keep your brochure or look at your website again. Thus, the ability to attract and focus your readers' attention and help them find specific information within your health promotion text becomes more and more important. This is especially true for extensive public health promotion brochures or websites that cover various subjects concerning a health topic, which may be relevant to readers at different times. So, for a brochure or website to be an effective help in changing behaviour or handling a disease, it should help guide the readers' attention as well as support selective reading.

Hence, knowing how people *use* health promotion materials may help effective design. More specifically, readers scan pages to get an impression of their contents or to find specific answers to their questions. Adjusting the materials' design to this scanning behaviour may facilitate readers in their search, but also help crucial messages that health promoters wish to convey, to stand out.

Learning Outcomes

After reading this chapter, you should be able to:

1 Analyse your health promotion materials in terms of their usability.
2 Design your health promotion materials in a user-friendly way.
3 Test the usability of your materials and identify potential improvements.

4.1 Usability

In cognitive psychological terms, 'usability' should be the focus in the design of information carriers, such as a brochure, website or leaflet. Usability is defined as 'the extent in which users of products are able to work *effectively*, *efficiently* and with *satisfaction*'. First, the effectiveness of a device refers to the extent to which a user can achieve specific goals by using it. Second, achieving a goal can occur more or less efficiently, depending on the user's expenditure of time or effort. Third, user-satisfaction concerns the perceived ease of use by users, so the subjective perception of how easy they found its use. Applied to written documents, a highly usable document would enable readers to locate information (effectiveness) with hardly any effort, so with minimal paging (efficiency), creating a positive attitude towards its contents, use and design (satisfaction). An additional effectiveness-related measure that is relevant to brochure design is its *learnability*, or the ease with which its contents and how to use it, are learned. So, in addition to thinking about what you wish to convey, you need to be aware of: (1) what readers want to know; and (2) how they will go about finding it in your materials. Involving members of your target group to study their responses to your draft materials can greatly improve them.

Studies that focus on how people typically use written documents can provide insights into how to adjust a document to its readers and by doing this, become more usable for them. For example, research has been done into how we can guide readers' attention through brochures and leaflets so that they can easily find specific information which they are looking for. These will be described in this chapter. Several usability criteria can aid you in designing or improving earlier designs for high(er) usability. Examples of good and bad design will illustrate our explanations, and we will describe easy ways to test the usability of preliminary document designs.

4.2 Attention processes: top-down and bottom-up

When thinking about your materials, you have identified their purpose and, based on this, you have made choices about the specific content you wish to convey. Advice on refining and crafting this content is provided in Chapters 6–10. At this stage, it may help to think about how your text will be read by considering both top-down (reader-initiated) and bottom-up (text-directed) influences on mental information processing. Figure 4.1 illustrates these influences.

'Top-down' refers to all processes (search processes as well as comprehension processes) that are generated by characteristics of the reader. These characteristics include the readers' prior experiences and knowledge, their mental capacities, but also the goal with which they open a brochure or access a website. Different knowledge and goals may trigger different expectations and with that, different reading or search strategies. Stated more simply for instance, readers who have some prior knowledge about a health-related subject may want to search for specific kinds of information in a brochure. For example, readers who know that their diet is less healthy and are wondering what healthy eating habits entail, will find explanations about calories in different kinds of food interesting to read.

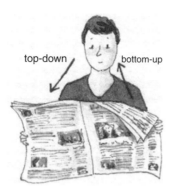

Figure 4.1   Top-down characteristics in the reader interact with bottom-up characteristics of the materials being read

However, readers who already know about their specific problem-areas concerning fatty foods, may want to find answers to practical issues about how to counter their tendency to buy these particular foods. Such people will selectively attend to, or search for the information they want, for instance for tips when going to the supermarket and healthy alternatives to their unhealthy preferences.

These top-down influences on text processing are based on the reader's prior experiences with a brochure's subject and with health promotion brochures in general. Based on this prior knowledge, readers may form expectations about what they are going to encounter in unfamiliar, new materials. This may help them to locate information in your materials. For example, readers may expect to encounter a table of contents on the first page and headings in the main text that signal the text's subjects on different text levels. The design of such features determines the text structure and thus the overview readers can attain when initially skimming through a brochure (Hartley, 2004, and see Chapter 1 in this book).

This latter example refers to a 'bottom-up' process, that is, an influence of the design elements on the reader. Visually distinguishing different kinds of information on a page or throughout a brochure may influence what relations readers perceive among those pieces of text. For instance, ensuring that headings of similar importance or text containing related information share the same type-size and colour may help readers understand that the subjects they introduce are of similar importance or similar in nature.

Top-down processes interact with bottom-up processes and may enhance or hinder each other. For example, depending on a reader's prior experience with using links in websites, they may feel more or less strongly invited to click on underlined pieces of text on screen. If the design of a website or brochure meets readers' expectations based on their prior knowledge, finding specific information will be easier. Because readers expect such features to help them find specific information, their presence in 'new' materials guides their attention as the text designer intended. However, unconventional design of text features may clash with the reader's expectations and result in sub-optimal processing of the information or, worse still, readers become lost in the text (see also Chapter 5).

When choosing an uncommon design format, an effort should be made to flag the structure of the information as well as how it should be used by readers, to make sure readers process the text as you expect and do not get lost.

As noted in the previous two chapters, an overview of text content and subject ordering helps readers find what they want. So, in terms of usability, an effective brochure is one in which the content structure is immediately clear when searching for information. If a designer wants readers to remember particular messages, these should be highlighted using 'access structures' such as a table of contents, topic headings, or an index, so they are easily located (Yussen et al., 1993). Including a clear table of contents with all headings ordered into main sections and sub-sections (i.e., a text's first, second, and third level) improve efficiency in locating desired information. Figure 4.2 illustrates such a table of contents.

4.3 Designing for usability

As we described above, enhancing usability means optimising the interaction between your readers' top-down processes and the bottom-up processing initiated by the design of your health promotion materials. As with understanding (see Chapter 3), knowing your readers is crucial. So ask yourself: Who is my target group? What do they know about the use of this type of materials? What questions will they have? How will they go about searching for answers to these questions? Knowing about readers' prior knowledge, expectations and mental processing habits will help you determine what messages are central and thus have to stand out, as well as which design elements will be helpful for your audience in finding what they are looking for.

Researchers who specialised in usability have defined a useful list of eight usability-criteria (Lin et al., 1997). These criteria are specific elements that add to effectiveness, efficiency, satisfaction and learnability. Although their research focused on websites, the criteria they formulated can also be applied to print materials, especially when they contain multiple pages through which readers need to navigate. These usability criteria can provide guidelines for testing preliminary drafts with your readers in later stages of the design process.

In short, a brochure or website design is more usable when:

1 stimulus-response compatibility is high;
2 it is internally and externally consistent;
3 it is flexible to the needs and wishes of various kinds of users;
4 it is easy to learn;
5 minimal action is required;
6 minimal working memory and long-term memory load are required;
7 considerations of limits in human perceptual organisation are embedded;
8 a user guidance scheme is available.

Writing health communication

CONTENTS

Figure 4.2   **A table of contents, designed into three groupings, each containing visually distinct sub-orderings. Notice how each hierarchical text level is made visually redundant, so graphically distinct from each other, in two ways: spacing, indentations from left and right, and type-sizes**

Making written materials easy to use

We will explain each criterion separately and provide examples of do's and don'ts, which are based on research into print as well as website design. Regarding website design we refer you to an excellent and very practical book called *Research-Based Web Design and Usability Guidelines*, by Leavitt and Schneiderman (2006).

Three things are important to be aware of before we go into details:

1   Especially with websites, where users can quickly click away from your website, applying the principles below is important to get your messages across.
2   Some of the tips below have multiple advantages and thus relate to multiple criteria at the same time. We only mention each tip once, with the criterion it has the strongest relation to.
3   Usable design is not necessarily a matter of applying all the examples below in one brochure or website. Each feature needs to be evaluated in relation to its effects in the context of the entire brochure or website as well as the type of audience you are designing your materials for.

When people want to find specific information, the usability of your brochure or website is important. You help your reader understand your design, find information fast and have a positive feeling about your materials, by applying the eight usability criteria just mentioned. These will be explained more thoroughly below.

4.3.1 Stimulus-response compatibility

The concept of response compatability means that there should be physical as well as conceptual correspondence between a stimulus and the reaction that it requires from the user. A button affords pushing it and invites more clearly when it stands out from its surrounding surface. In this example, there is a physical correspondence between the stimulus (the button) and the response (pushing it). A picture of a button in a website, that you can click on with the mouse, is a conceptual translation from the real-time, physical correspondence between stimulus and action. Thus, any graphical element in a text or website that literally mimics the 'use' of its real-time equivalent, is conceptually compatible and therefore provokes user-actions. Note that they may also *hinder* usability if they are implemented the wrong way. For example, underlined words on screen are conceptually seen as 'links' on which you can click to go to related information. Underlining important words in your web-text without creating links at those places will annoy readers who wish to use them that way.

So, what helps and what does not help? Some examples are given below:

Do
In a brochure:

• Use arrows to point to related pieces of text that you wish readers to associate with each other.

Writing health communication

- Use tabs that stick out from the pages, so that readers can grab them and use them to flip to information flagged by the tab.

On a website:

- Use underlining and blue coloration for text, or icons and pictures to invite users to click and be linked to related information.

Don't
In a brochure:

- Place text belonging to a tab on the page that the tab is attached to. Users will use the tab to turn over the page, expecting the information to be behind, not on the same page as the tab.

On a website:

- Ensure that items that are not clickable do not have characteristics that suggest that they are clickable. Bullets and arrows may suggest clickability even when they contain no other clickability cues.

4.3.2 Internal and external consistency

With this we mean that the layout of each page should be the same as the layout of the other pages which in turn, should match that of other health promotion brochures or websites. This has to do with general expectations that readers have, based on their previous experience with brochures and websites as well as their specific expectations that you cause readers to form when they open your brochure or enter your website. For instance, readers expect some overview of the brochure contents on the first page as well as similar headings to indicate similar text levels. On a website, users expect a homepage from which they can navigate to all main sections or subpages in a similar manner. So, be consistent in your choices and follow them through throughout your design.

Do
In a brochure:

- Flag different text levels with graphically similar headings, in colour as well as font-size and spacing.
- Use similar page-layouts throughout the entire brochure, so that readers don't have to find out how to read each page again.
- If you make an important message stand out, for instance, in bold or in the margin of the page, do so with all the messages that need to stand out.

On a website:

- Repeat your entire navigation bar on top and to the left of each page.
- Provide a search option on each page.
- Use the colours, possibly your brand colours, which your readers will recognise.

Making written materials easy to use

Don't

In a brochure:

- Make each new page a piece of art. This may be a graphical designer's dream, but in general, artistic novelties need second and third glances for readers and annoy those who are distracted by content-free graphics.

On a website:

- Change the location of your navigation bar on different web pages throughout one website.

4.3.3 Flexibility

The term flexibility means that your interface should be able to adapt to users' needs. Different users may have different needs due to different levels of skill and their needs may change over time as well because they improve their skills. Applying this criterion to websites may be more straightforward than to written materials, which in the end can only be paged through. However, when applied to brochures that contain multiple kinds of information, flexibility can be thought of as a navigational system that affords jumping from subject to subject without having to return to the contents page every time.

Do

In a brochure:

- Insert overviews of important subjects with page numbers on each page, possibly accompanied by the statement 'related subjects you may wish to read in this brochure'.
- Use many headings that cover the text contents well, so that readers can visually 'jump' easily from subject to subject.
- Insert tabs that afford jumping from one section to another, in a forward direction as well as back to previous subjects.

On a website:

- Enable users to customise window attributes, such as font, size of the window, foreground and background colours, etc.
- Make sure that important links are provided on each page, no matter how 'deep' users are in your website.
- Make links within your website redundant, so place them at multiple places even on the same page. This redundancy creates a fail-safe, with which you make sure that important links are found regardless of coincidence.
- Provide information in multiple formats if your website has distinct audiences who will be interested in the same information, for instance, with separate links for 'the public', 'practitioners' and 'researchers'. This allows you to provide several levels of technical details according to the needs of these audiences.

Don't

In a brochure:

- Make the text too fragmented with your headings; you need to strike a balance between segmentation and unity with the use of your headings.

On a website:

- Place a link only once on the homepage and nowhere else. Once users have clicked away from the homepage, they may not return.

4.3.4 Learnability

Good design is easy to learn. The learning process will be enhanced through a clear and well-organised layout or interface. Central for learnable design is the issue of whether it makes sense to your audience. In other words: are the design choices you made logical from your audience's perspective? In deciding upon information ordering, keep in mind that when the textual structure is in agreement with readers' expectations, text processing and learning are facilitated. Narratives in our culture typically have a basic exposition–complication–resolution structure. Maintaining this structure will aid comprehension and learnability. Note too that following the advice in the previous chapter, on text comprehension, and in Chapters 6 and 7 of this book will also enhance the learnability of the contents of your materials.

Do

In a brochure:

- Order subjects in a logical order, applying a cause-to-effect, or an exposition–complication–resolution structure on all text levels throughout your materials.
- Make each change in text subject explicit, with clear headings that cover the content of the paragraph.
- Use attention-attracting features with caution and only when they are highly relevant.

On a website:

- Order menu options according to their: functionality; expected frequency of use; alphabetic ordering.
- Be consistent in the way you arrange your navigational tools, regarding their placement as well as their design.
- Make the grouping and the ordering of menu options logical.
- Choose meaningful command names.

Making written materials easy to use

Don't

In a brochure:

- Use headings that may be catchy but difficult to relate to the text they are supposed to cover.

On a website:

- Use dynamic elements that keep moving on screen; they distract the readers' attention away from the contents of a webpage.

4.3.5 Minimal action

This fifth usability criterion states that users should only have to perform a minimal number of actions to finish a task with your materials. Specifically, when they are looking up specific information, they should be able to do so with minimal paging and scanning, or with minimal clicking, scrolling and scanning.

Do

In a brochure:

- Make sure readers can go to the section of interest by paging only once, for instance, from the contents page onward. This means paying extra attention to clear and structured headings in a clear contents page

On a website:

- Keep your website only three levels 'deep'. The more clicks that are needed to get to information, the smaller the chance that your audience will get there. So, make sure minimal steps are required for menu selection.
- Put the most important messages on the first and second levels of your web-site, that is, on the home-page and manually one click further on.
- Make sure that minimal cursor positioning is necessary.
- Keep running text restricted in length, so that no scrolling is necessary. Insert a 'home' link on every page in exactly the same location.
- If readers need to scroll down to read text, repeat the 'home' and 'back' button on the bottom of the page.

Don't

On a website:

- Put singular links or buttons below screen view; users should not have to scroll to be able to see them.

Writing health communication

4.3.6 Minimal working memory and long-term memory load

The less users need to keep in mind or learn about how to use your materials, the faster they will learn it. Thus, making navigation and conceptual links visible for users will help them to learn how to use your brochure or website.

Do
In a brochure:

- Introduce a system that invites readers to put their questions, thoughts or remarks near the piece of text that triggered those ideas.
- Use a minimum of abbreviations or acronyms.
- Provide supplementary verbal labels for icons.

On a website:

- Make the guidance and help information always available.
- Provide hierarchic menus for sequential selection.
- Highlight selected links.
- Make a 'breadcrumb trail', showing the sequence of clicks made by the user.
- Use short words for links and buttons.
- Partition long data-entries, for instance, for a phone number entry.

4.3.7 Limits to human perceptual organisation

The term 'perceptual organisation' refers to the way people understand relationships among separate elements in your materials. For example, the principles of 'Gestalt' describe how separate elements in a visual display may be perceived as a group, or as belonging together. To understand how to apply Gestalt principles in texts, have another look at the table of contents in Figure 4.2, shown earlier. This table of contents was designed according to general principles of perceptual grouping, which emanate from the *Gestalt principles of 'precedence', 'symmetry', and 'enclosure'* (see, for instance, Winn, 1994). That is, with spacing of headings and indentations of headings that share the same text level, the design attempts to create visually evident groupings of sections, thus enhancing the ease of scanning the contents page. The three levels in the brochure text were indicated typographically. This was done in at least two ways simultaneously, making the structure of the brochure visually salient and thus easily recognisable. For example, the three main section titles were highlighted with bold capital letters, which stood out from the remaining lower case normal lettering of the sub-headings. To emphasise that there were three main sections, the three groups of headings of each section were separated by a white line, creating three 'blocks' of text. Dotted lines that linked the page numbers to their headings, added to the visual perception of these 'blocks'. To highlight the three levels of headings in the brochure, the headings on each lower level were indented one tab and made one type-size smaller. This way, all headings that were on the same level were

Making written materials easy to use

on the same indentation on the page and the same, unique size. A third feature that distinguished the two lowest levels of headings was the indentation of the page numbers on the right side of the page. So, with typographical cueing the table of contents was structurally arranged to enable readers to perceive and remember the information hierarchy of the brochure. Lastly, the entire table of contents was fitted on one page, to ensure a full overview of the contents in one glance.

To summarise:

Do
In brochures as well as on websites:

- Put related text subjects close together on a page (principle of proximity).
- Put text and pictures belonging to the text close together (principle of proximity).
- Give related text subjects similar form, colour and orientation (principle of similarity).
- Use vertical and horizontal spacing around text blocks and pictures you want readers to see as units.
- Use the same colour or grey-scale to signal elements that belong together.
- Display a series of related items in a vertical list rather than as continuous text. This facilitates rapid and accurate scanning.

Don't
In brochures as well as on websites:

- Use green and red to signal two distinct subjects; colour-blindness prevents a group of people perceiving the difference between these colours.
- Use colours with little contrast in saturation close together; some readers may not perceive the difference.

4.3.8 User guidance scheme

A brochure or website which contains a good user guidance scheme will help readers navigate through the information. This, in turn, will improve the material's learnability, as well as decrease mental workload for users and possibly the number of actions they need to perform while using it. A good user guidance scheme will reduce memory load so the do's and don'ts mentioned in section 4.3.6 are relevant here as well.

Do
In a brochure:

- Make sure that on each page it is clear to your readers where in the brochure they are. For instance, you can do this with the list of subjects on top or in the margin of each page, with the relevant section highlighted.

- Indicate separate kinds of information, so that readers know on first glance whether pages contain for instance background information, specific details, action-related or to-do information.
- Include a short section at the start, on the contents page, for instance, which tells the readers how to use your brochure. It might indicate which sections of information are important and which actions related to that text should be read after that.

On a website:

- Provide clear system feedback when users make mistakes, for instance, with erroneous entries in a 'search' option of your website. Make the error message helpful, with tips on what kinds of entries are expected.
- Use location and highlighting to prioritise pushbuttons, with the most-used pushbutton in the first position.

4.4 How to apply the above usability criteria: an example

By now you may feel overwhelmed with tips for usable designs. Let's make it clearer by adding an example of how to apply the 'dos' we described. Figures 4.3(a) and 4.3(b) provide an illustration of how the usability criteria described above were applied to evaluate and improve a brochure (for details, see Kools et al., 2007).

With the eight usability criteria above in mind, we analysed this brochure and identified a number of usability problems. Throughout the brochure, short paragraphs were inserted to highlight related text. These looked similar to the contents page shown in Figure 4.3a in that they were accompanied by the same arrow-pictorial and mentioned a subsequent page that readers should go to. However, these reference-paragraphs were of variable lengths and were placed at variable places throughout the brochure. This lowered their *internal consistency*. In addition, use of reference paragraphs throughout the text is rather unconventional, so readers could not rely on prior experience in using them (thus causing low *external consistency*).

In another study, the arrow-pictorial that accompanied these sections had been shown to be unclear to readers (see Chapter 3). Therefore, this pictorial was *lowering external consistency*. This, in turn could result in low recognition and poor use of the pictorial to identify useful subsequent pages (that is, *low stimulus-response compatibility*). Referring readers to other sections that could be relevant for them is an attempt to enhance the flexibility with which the brochure can be used, but readers have to have read the previous text first before being directed to another section. So these reference paragraphs are not enabling readers to use the text in individualised ways. Instead they determine a single storyline resulting in *low flexibility*. Given that the brochure contained a lot of information without a complete contents page on which the information hierarchy was presented, we

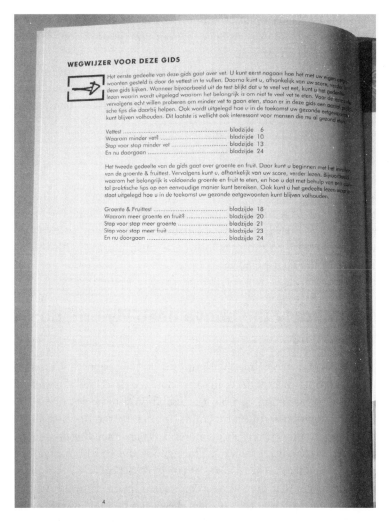

Figure 4.3(a)   Picture of the original brochure

expected that learning its general contents was relatively difficult (low *learnability* of brochure content). In addition, a higher-than-necessary *minimal amount of action* was required to find specific information elements. Altogether, although an attempt was made to design a *user guidance scheme*, the design of this brochure and its guidance system was sub-optimal in terms of usability.

Based on this analysis, an adjusted version of the original brochure was designed, which is shown in Figure 4.3(b).

To improve the brochure's access structures and usability a combination of three changes was made: tabs were inserted, the original brochure's arrows were replaced by conventional arrows and colour-coding was applied to the combination of arrows and tabs. In terms of usability, the tabs were expected to have high *external consistency* because they are also typically encountered in address books or office books as

Writing health communication

Figure 4.3(b) An adjusted version of the brochure in Figure 4.3(a), adjusted according to the eight usability guidelines described in the text (See the colour section at the end of the book)

aids for accessibility. The tabs were made maximally visible by extending them from the right side of the page, thus showing users where they are in the brochure at all times. This would add to *user guidance*. In addition, the tabs gave users an overview of the brochure's contents, improving potential *learnability* of its main contents. Related to this, the clarity of the three main subjects was enhanced by grouping the tabs of each main section together and leaving openings between each cluster of tabs (high *perceptual organisation*). The colour-coding of the tabs and arrows was designed to add to this grouping effect. Furthermore, the presence of the tabs was expected to decrease users' necessary *memory load*, as they did not need to remember page-numbers and names of headings when looking something up. In addition, the tabs could be picked up individually and so, by themselves, were expected to

Making written materials easy to use

afford page turning (providing high *stimulus-response compatibility*) while also lowering the required *minimal action* needed to find information. The tabs were expected to sustain the referencing-sections as well as function as a general table of contents for users, thus adding to the brochure's *flexibility* for readers with different needs.

> Implementing the above criteria in ways that we describe, will make your health promotion brochure or website more user-friendly.

Less skilled readers are expected to benefit even more than highly skilled readers from the presence of these signals on how to read and use your text. That is, readers with less skill may not be able to find the information at all in a brochure without clear access structures such as a table of contents and main section heading.

Finally, we strongly advise you to test your materials with the target audience to ensure they are used and understood as you intend. As design specialists we may feel confident about our choices but our intuitions may prove deceptive. Confidence in design skills is one of the major reasons that health education materials are not pilot-tested (Gal and Prigat, 2004). So remember, especially when you include uncommon features, you should test your designs and their effects on usability. The remainder of this chapter will tell you how to go about this, depending on what you aim for with your design choices.

4.5 How to test for usability

After designing your materials with their usability in mind, you, yourself, can check for usability on the eight criteria above. Based on that, you may initially make some adjustments. However, you will only know for certain about the effects of your choices on readers, when observing *them* while using your materials.

When observing readers, it is important to know what you want to know about the usability of the brochure. The decisions made in the design phase of the development process may help in forming a coding scheme of which behaviours should be recorded. For example, you may want some kinds of information to get most of the readers' attention and intend particular elements to help readers navigate the material according to their interests. In addition to the observational data, readers' subjective evaluations of accessibility and usability may generate ideas for improvements of your design. Subjective measures can indicate users' satisfaction with the materials, which may highlight changes that need to be made. But remember they may be reluctant to criticise!

4.5.1 Sample size

How much work does this pre-testing involve? Experimental comparisons between different versions of a design with 20–25 persons per group are required to enable scientifically reliable conclusions with regard to the effects of your design. Keep in mind here that even small differences that are found between such groups, for instance, in the speed in which they can find information, may reflect significant differences in cognitive demands which may have important real-world effects on the use of your materials (Wright, 1999).

If groups this size cannot be tested due to time or cost constraints, it is still worth conducting smaller tests. Small-scale pre-testing relies on qualitative data arising from assessments of participants' answers to comprehension questions or questions on particular text or visual elements. Having participants look up information while thinking aloud can identify difficulties in materials and potential misinterpretations. Research has shown that performing such 'user trials' with only four or five people may reveal up to 80 per cent of all potential usability problems with a design (Virzi, 1992). Thus, at relatively little cost, poor design of health promotion materials can be prevented. Each of the four aspects of usability – effectiveness, efficiency, satisfaction and learnability – may result in different test questions and tasks. Below, we explore the kinds of questions that can be asked.

4.5.2 Effectiveness

Here the central question is: 'Do my design choices have the effects I intended?' For instance: 'Does the information I want to stand out, indeed draw readers' attention?', 'Do people use the contents page and find information from it?', 'Are my pictures noticed and associated with the accompanying text?', 'Do people use the tabs in the way I intended?' Visual attention can be measured by measuring eye-movement patterns. Commercial companies have specialised in tracking eye-movements and use of booklets. These fixation patterns can be very informative. For instance, research into readers' eye-fixation patterns (Hyönä and Lorch, 2004) showed that readers' first-pass fixation time and the average look-back fixation time were notably longer towards topic headings than towards other text regions. This reflects the function of topic headings as facilitators of text processing, resulting in better memory for text topics. Such data may help you as a designer to check which features on each page draw most attention. Linking the results with other information regarding usability and learning indicates whether or not textual elements are as effective as expected. For example, if readers don't remember a certain slogan, this may be explained by another feature on the same page drawing their visual attention away from the key message.

Asking people to undertake tasks such as finding information or asking comprehension questions, watching how they do this and interviewing them about their experience will provide insights into the effectiveness of navigational features in your leaflet, brochure or website. You may measure the timing of their progress and count the errors they make. Doing this with two versions of your brochure shows you which one is the more usable. An additional important question is whether information is remembered or learned, which we discuss below.

4.5.3 Learnability: recall of the structure

Learning here has two dimensions: readers learning how to use your materials and readers learning the main messages you wish to convey (see also Chapter 3).

The more usable your design is, the easier it will be to learn its contents and how to navigate through it. Questions you may ask include: 'Do people get an overview of the brochure or website contents after they have used it?', 'Do they recall the main messages?', 'Do they have an insight into the ordering of the messages?'

If a health promotion text is intended as reference guide, readers should be able to recall the document's main themes so that they know how to use it when they return to it. Recalling its overall structure will help them find answers to new questions. For this, they need a mental representation of the textual structure. For example, you may want readers to understand a brochure's macrostructure, or the main themes as indicated with section and paragraph headings. When initially reading, skimming through, or looking up specific information, this division into main and subsections is important to building up a mental representation of the brochure's content.

Several measures tap into this superficial, usability-related understanding:

1 *Open recall questions*. Immediately after the initial paging-through, these questions test users' memory of the brochure's main structure, with questions such as: 'Can you tell me what the main sections were that the brochure consists of?' When you find that a particular section is forgotten, you could ask a second question, probing the user's memory further. Observations may provide you with insights into why mistakes are made.

2 *Flesch index*. Any Word-editor can calculate the Flesch readability score for your texts. This test calculates the ratio between the average sentence-length and the average number of syllables per word, thus providing a score between 0 and 100, showing how easy it is to read your text.

3 *Cloze-index*. This is another readability measure. Take out every fifth word from a piece of text and have users fill those in while reading. Calculating the ratio between correct words and mistakes will give you an indication of how 'readable' and thus understandable your text is. This measure has two advantages compared to the Flesch index: first, it includes actual users and thus their prior knowledge about the text subject, which is, as explained in Chapter 3, crucial to text understanding. Second, it provides straightforward clues on how to improve your text, namely at the places that readers made mistakes.

4 *Card sorting task*. To gain insight into the overview readers have gained after using your brochure or website, you can give them a set of cards with several text subjects and ask them to order them in the way they think the brochure or website was ordered. You can ask them to show the text levels, e.g., main and sub-sections. You can assess the quality of the users' sorting in several ways, depending on your interests. For instance, how many and which labels did they remember regarding the main sections? Also, errors can be counted in their recall of the sub-sections within the main sections. The order may be of interest as well as the *number of intrusions* of sub-headings into wrong main sections. Using sorting cards is

Writing health communication

easier for readers than recalling the structure. If different readers consistently fail to order topics as they are presented in the text, this may suggest that the text ordering does not correspond to readers' perceptual or logical organisation of the subject matter – and could imply that re-ordering is needed to enhance learnability.

4.5.4 Efficiency

Efficiency refers to the ease with which users reach their goals using your materials. Whether they find answers to their questions is a matter of effectiveness; *how fast* they can do so has to do with efficiency. Low efficiency may cause low effectiveness because when it takes users too long to find what they are looking for, they stop searching and do not reach their goal. So it is difficult to measure effectiveness and efficiency separately. In our study into the usability of the brochure shown in Figures 4.3a and 4.3b, participants were asked; 'Where in the brochure does the section about fruit and vegetables start?', 'Where does it give tips on how to maintain eating changes, when you cook the food yourself?', and 'Where is it explained what to do, to prevent eating fatty snacks between meals?' Each time, the time they needed to locate that specific information and the number of pages they turned before finding the answers, were measured. Search efficiency was defined as the time needed to locate search items and the amount of paging through the brochure before the answers were found. The more pages that had to be turned and scanned, the less efficient was the search. We found lower paging frequency in the group with the adjusted brochure compared to the original, which indicated that users of the modified brochure were able to use a more efficient, selective search strategy.

4.5.5 Satisfaction

Finally, your brochure or website may be effective, efficient and learnable but if it does not meet the needs of your target audience, it will not have the impact you aimed for. The extent to which readers find it interesting and attractive may be just as important to its impact as the usability measures above. Just ask your readers what they think about several features you are interested in. You can do this with a questionnaire or a short interview. Being face-to-face with users can help in enabling them to be more critical (especially if you distance yourself from the design and describe it as a prototype) and may provide greater insight into the reasons underlying their evaluation of the materials. Open general questions such as 'Is there anything in the brochure you particularly like or dislike?' are useful starting points. You could also ask for their opinions of the graphical elements or guage their liking of several elements on a 10-point like–dislike response scale. During such testing, we have, for example, found that readers preferred many headings and relatively high segmentation of text.

4.6 Conclusion

Making the usability of your health promotion materials central to your design can enhance their impact. Thinking in terms of usability is thinking about your readers' visual attention or perceptual processes, about cognitive processes underlying their interpretation of your interventions, and finally, thinking about the actions or actual handling of your materials by your readers. Usability is about making your 'users' or audience central in the design process. So, ask yourself three basic questions. First: 'What goals will readers have, what do they want to know or learn?'. Second: 'How does this fit with my goals, or the messages I want to convey to them?'. And third: 'What kind of information carrier and which design elements will be effective in conveying these messages?' This chapter then, provides tips and guidelines to help you make these choices as well as test their effects.

References

Gal, I. and Prigat, A. (2004) 'Why organizations continue to create patient information leaflets with readability and usability problems: an explorative study', *Health Education Research Advance Access*, Dec. 21.

Hartley, J. (2004) 'Designing instructional and informational text', in D.H. Jonassen (ed.), *Handbook of Research on Educational Communication and Technology*. Mahwah, NJ: Erlbaum, pp. 917–47.

Hyöna, J. and Lorch, R.F. (2004) 'Effects of topic headings on text processing: evidence from adult readers' eye fixation patterns', *Learning and Instruction*, 14: 131–52.

Kools, M., Ruiter, R.A.C., Van de Wiel, M.W.J., and Kok, G. (2007) 'Testing the usability of access structures in a health education brochure', *British Journal of Health Psychology*, 12: 525–41.

Leavitt, O. and Schneiderman, B. (2006) *Research-Based Web Design and Usability Guidelines*. Washington, DC: U.S. Government Printing Office.

Lin, H.X., Choong, Y.Y. and Salvendy, G. (1997) 'A proposed index of usability: a method for comparing the relative usability of different software systems', *Behaviour and Information Technology*, 16: 267–78.

Virzi, R.A. (1992) 'Refining the test phase of usability evaluation: how many subjects is enough?' *Human Factors*, 34: 457–68.

Winn, W. (1994) 'Contributions of perceptual and cognitive processes to the comprehension of graphics', in W. Schnotz and R.W. Kulhavy (eds), *Comprehension of Graphics*. Amsterdam: North-Holland, pp. 3–27.

Wright, P. (1999) 'Designing healthcare advice for the public', in F.T. Durso, R.S. Nickerson, R.W. Schvaneveldt, S.T. Dumais, D.S. Lindsay and M.T.H. Chi (eds), *Handbook of Applied Cognition*. New York: John Wiley & Sons Ltd, pp. 396–460.

Yussen, S.R., Stright, A.D. and Payne, B. (1993) 'Where is it? Searching for information in a college textbook', *Contemporary Educational Psychology*, 18: 240–57.

5

Using graphics effectively in text

Patricia Wright

As we saw in Chapter 3, if graphics are to help people reading about healthcare, choices of graphic styles and location within documents must suit the intended communicative purpose of the graphic. For example, wrong choices can disadvantage older readers because the graphics distract them from the main message. This chapter explains how to make the right choices and has three main sections. The first discusses the different functions graphics can have in health materials. The second highlights what you need to bear in mind when selecting among graphic styles: *Will a line drawing be sufficient or is a colour photograph needed?* Finally, the third section outlines the problems that can arise, and the design trade-offs that may be needed, when fitting graphics onto a page: *To keep everything on the same page, would it be better to have a bigger picture and smaller text or vice versa?*

For convenience this chapter will focus on printed materials, often using the label 'leaflets' as a shorthand for the diversity of healthcare information which includes labels on medicines and notices on clinic walls and guidance booklets; but the advice is based on principles from research on how people attend, read and understand. These principles have wide applicability and are relevant to the design of online text. You may find it helpful to think of the underlying structure of this chapter as a matrix in which the communication purposes outlined in Section 5.1 need to be related to the choices of graphic styles discussed in Section 5.2.

Learning Outcomes

After reading this chapter, you should be able to:

1. Understand the different purposes graphics can serve in healthcare materials.
2. Recognise where you can use graphics to help readers find, understand and remember information.
3. Know how to avoid the common pitfalls when using drawings, photographs or data charts.
4. Be able to select graphic styles to meet your communication purposes.
5. Know how to make design trade-offs when integrating graphics and text.
6. Understand the importance of pilot testing your graphics in the full context of your leaflet.

5.1 Why include graphics?

Graphics can help readers in several ways. For example, graphics helped patients who had undergone heart surgery understand the need for participation in a cardiac rehabilitation programme, when their doctor used a line drawing of the heart and arteries to show where and how much the patient's arteries were occluded. Discussion with other patients indicated it was rare for doctors to use graphics in this way, although many other patients commented that they too would have found it very helpful (Osborne, 2006). Yet the tendency not to provide graphics is widespread. When adults gave written directions for crossing a town centre from A to B very few people included a map or diagram, although most of these people chose a style that included some form of graphic when selecting directions they would like to use themselves (Wright et al., 1995). Perhaps writers forget to use graphics because they write in the same way that they would tell someone if they were talking to them or because they doubt their own artistic abilities. Both these lines of thinking need to be resisted because graphics can be very helpful.

5.1.1 Good advice exists

Patient information leaflets that accompany medicines contain illustrations such as line drawings showing actions to be taken, realistic coloured photographs, abstract diagrams depicting processes, statistical charts, and cartoons. With such a range, it is no surprise that graphics have the potential both to enlighten and to confuse. Yet good advice on using graphics abounds. The following six guidelines for graphics in healthcare information are derived from principles proposed by Kosslyn (2006):

1   The most important information being conveyed should correspond to the illustration's most striking visual features because these will capture the reader's attention.
2   The design of graphics must encourage readers to make the intended groupings of visual items and also foster the appropriate spatial or temporal organisation of the message elements.
3   The visual appearance of the graphic needs to be compatible with meaning, e.g. the direction 'up' means *greater* or *improving*, not *worse*; people find positives (e.g. *more*) easier to understand than negatives (e.g. *less*). The information given in the graphic must be neither too much, where the details may obscure the message, nor too little, where the result may be an inadequate or shallow understanding of the message, which in turn can lead to non-adherence to the information.
4   The design of the graphic must take account of the knowledge, or lack of it, that readers will have, especially their familiarity with the concepts, jargon and symbols that are used to convey the message.
5   The graphic conventions used throughout a leaflet should be consistent but if an exception is necessary, e.g. to give a close-up view, these changes should be clearly signalled to avoid misinterpretation.

5.1.2 Good advice Is not enough

Most people are happy to agree with the above advice but much patient information is poor (Raynor et al., 2007). Will your own leaflet conform to these principles? As has been emphasised in Chapters 2 and 3, often pilot testing is the only way to check that your intended meaning reaches readers. Following good advice increases your chances that this will be the case but cannot guarantee it because so many factors interact to influence the success of a specific graphic. It helps writers if they have a framework for thinking about design issues.

One simple framework is to think of designing graphics for leaflets as a three-stage process:

1   decide on the purpose of the graphic;
2   select a graphic style;
3   locate the graphics appropriately within the leaflet.

This linear sequence is an oversimplification. When the text is seen on the page, the graphic may need to be resized to fit the available space, but the illustration (e.g. a photograph) may not communicate well at the new size (e.g. if shrunk). So at the *'location'* stage (3) the previous decision about graphic style may need to be revisited, and a photograph replaced with an outline drawing that can be fitted into the space. Nevertheless, these three stages are reflected in the following sections because thinking about each stage will alert you to potential pitfalls when using graphics.

5.2 Stage 1: what is the purpose of your graphic?

Graphics can serve purposes that range from giving information to providing amusement. Being clear about the reason for using a graphic is the first step towards selecting an appropriate graphic style and locating that graphic appropriately on the page. Of course a single graphic can serve more than one purpose, but that is not a reason for ignoring what those purposes are. In this section we will consider four common functions of graphics:

1   attracting people to read the leaflet;
2   helping readers locate the information they want;
3   clarifying explanations given in the text, especially helping people understand numerical concepts such as probability and risk;
4   helping readers carry out procedures that are mentioned in the text.

Start by thinking about the various places in your leaflet where you could incorporate graphics to help your readers use the information and also help your message to get across.

5.2.1 Using graphics to attract readers

Leaflets available in public places, such as doctors' waiting rooms, need to attract readers to the information. The topic of the leaflet will encourage some people pick it up, but healthcare leaflets can also be intended for those who do not know or do not care about the topic. For this audience, design can be very influential. Improvements to nutrition labels were found to be most effective for people with little interest in healthy eating (Black and Rayner, 1992), perhaps because those people who cared about their diet were willing to make more effort to understand the poorer designs. If the images on a leaflet's cover correspond to a particular ethnic group, this helps members of that group identify with the message of the leaflet (Springston and Champion, 2004). On the other hand, a leaflet about drug taking that was intended for a teenage audience was ignored by many American teenagers. Some thought the illustrations suggested the information was intended for a younger age group, others felt that the people shown (and hence the message) were from decades past (Schriver, 1997, p. 173). So the wrong image on the cover can undermine the leaflet.

In many everyday contexts, people are reluctant readers. When 327 people responded to a questionnaire given to them as they left a doctor's waiting room in the UK, only 20 people said they had read any of the leaflets that were available on a table in the waiting room or notices on the walls (Wicke et al., 1994). The reasons for this reluctance to read can include poor literacy and numeracy skills, and also emotional stress. Graphics can dispel the appearance of a leaflet being 'heavy' reading. Similarly, graphics can change the mental picture of the author that people create as they read. Even on a tax form, including photographs of potential official contacts not only made the form seem more attractive and less discouraging but also made the form-fillers feel more positive towards the tax department (van Wijk and Arts, 2008).

The need for an appealing design also applies to the layout within a leaflet. Chapter 3 showed how layout can enhance readers' ease of understanding the message. The 'at a glance' visual appearance of pages can also change the tone of a leaflet, making the information seem friendlier or livelier. This is illustrated in the contrast between the two layouts shown in Figure 5.1. On the left of Figure 5.1 is a page of text having the visual style of an official letter or notice. The version on the right uses space graphically, varies the fonts, and changes the number of columns within the notice from single column above the box to double column below the box, reflecting the different status of the information. The main message is enclosed in a box centred on the page. Graphically this tells readers: *If you do not want to read everything, just read this.* The resulting layout falls between the genres adopted by magazines and posters. This was done deliberately so that readers would not dismiss it as being '*just another X*'. No word of the text content was changed, only the visual impact of the page and thereby the response it elicits from readers.

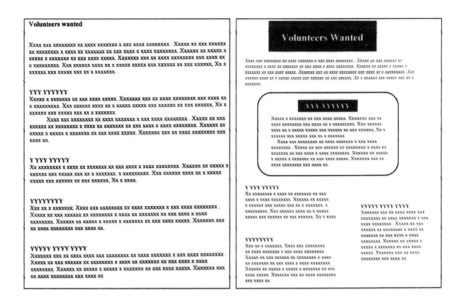

Figure 5.1 Two ways of laying out the same content. If you were sitting in a waiting room, which of the two would you read first?

Check how your readers respond to the appearance of your leaflet:

1   Will the cover image attract the intended audience?
2   Inside the leaflet, is it friendly or formal? Does its appearance make it look as though it will be easy or hard to read? Do people want to start reading it now or wait until later?

5.2.2 Graphics can help people find information

Even though an explanation may be clear in words (e.g. *Drinking this will make you ill*), a small graphic (e.g. a first aid sign) alongside the text, to identify the topic or the relevant audience, can increase the chance that this information within the leaflet will be read. The use of graphic organisers is illustrated in Chapter 3 but small graphics in page headers or margins can also serve an incidental '*you are here*' sign-posting function. Such graphics need to be easily identifiable and clearly distinguished from each other. People can often scan graphic images looking for a particular target faster than they scan through words; repeating the same graphic too often (e.g. in the header of every page) can potentially undermine this purpose of pinpointing target information.

It is not being suggested that leaflets should include spurious graphics just to provide visual landmarks. On the contrary, some readers, e.g. people over 70 years, can be distracted by graphics that have only a very general relation to the topic, although these same readers were not affected by explanatory illustrations (Griffin and Wright, 2008). Perhaps all the graphics were potentially distracting

Using graphics effectively in text

for older people, but the appropriate graphics had benefits that compensated for this. In order to make graphics work for you, you need to be clear about what work you want them to do.

Points you need to check:

1 Are your graphics easily distinguishable from each other?
2 Do your graphics add to the information content, rather than just make the page look pretty?
3 Will your graphics help readers find the information they are looking for?

5.2.3 Graphics can support explanations

Graphics can amplify details from the text, removing ambiguities about the direction of an action or the location of internal parts of the body. Graphics are not constrained by the linearity of sentence structures, so they can help readers understand dynamic biological processes such as the digestive tract or circulatory system or muscle movements where several processes occur at the same time but have interdependencies. Chapter 3 illustrates how explanatory diagrams can be used. In contrast, this section will discuss graphics that explain risk, tables that can help readers understand contextual dependencies (*If this ..., then that ...*), and maps that explain how you can get from A to B.

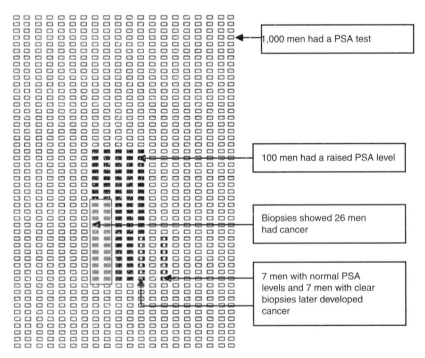

Figure 5.2   **An example of how text and graphics can be combined to explain complex information – *if this is your PSA level, then that is your likelihood of cancer***

Writing health communication

Not everyone is comfortable with numerical concepts, and some people may not understand nutrition information or blood pressure levels or medication dosages. It is known that explaining the risk of side-effects from medication using words such as *common* or *rare*, results in people tending to overestimate the level of harm from taking the medication. People thought '*common*' was closer to '*certain*' than was intended, and *rare* was thought to mean '*it could happen*' rather than '*it is unlikely to happen*' (Knapp et al., 2004). Understanding improves when probabilities are expressed as frequencies, e.g. *three people in a thousand rather than 0.3 per cent* (Gigerenzer and Hoffrage, 1995). Further advantage can come from showing these frequencies pictorially (Edwards et al., 2007). Figure 5.2 illustrates the likely outcomes from a screening test for prostate cancer, a test that is widely used but misses some cancers (false negatives) and mistakenly flags some people as possibly having cancer (false positives). An animated graphic explaining these risks can be seen at www.prosdex.com.

Of course not all numeric information requires pictures. Simple tables may suffice, for example, showing the relation between patient age and medicine dose. Similarly not all tables require numbers. Tables giving explanations are often textual. An example is given in Figure 5.3 where the links between cause and effect are explained in a trouble-shooting context.

Fault	Possible Cause	Action needed
Machine not working	Cover not securely closed	• Close cover
	Pilot light not glowing	• Check machine is switched on • Check if fuse has blown
	Start lever is up	• Push start lever down
No water in machine	Infill hose is blocked or disconnected	• Check infill hose
	Water not turned on	• Turn on water

Figure 5.3   The lines and space make it clear which items belong together

One of the common mistakes when designing tables is to put lines around every cell. This stops readers visually grasping which items belong together; instead people have to work this out from the content. In Figure 5.3 horizontal lines emphasise the relation between the causes of problems and their cures. The same visual grouping could have been achieved by the use of space or colour rather than lines. The important design factor is to create an appropriate 'at a glance' visual grouping; the way this is achieved matters much less.

A different kind of explanation that can benefit from graphics arises when you need to explain how to find specific clinics or offices within a large building. Then it is helpful to provide a diagram, floor plan or map that people can have with them as they travel to their destination (Wright et al. 1993). Readers will use this

Using graphics effectively in text

for reference and turn to it for information and reassurance. If there is scale variation within the graphic (e.g. to shorten a long corridor) this needs to be clearly indicated. Including landmarks within the graphic, especially at choice points, enhances its usefulness. These landmarks might be provided by architectural features, e.g. turn right just beyond the window (or notice board, etc.) or they may be other graphic features such as floor pattern or wall colour. Whatever feature is selected as a landmark needs to be salient on the graphic aid people are given.

Explaining how to do something can be much the same as instructing them in what to do (see Section 5.1) especially if there is little choice involved, but diagrams, maps and floor plans can support explanatory as well as instructional purposes. For example, by showing the problems with a specific route, visual representations graphically explain why another route is preferable. Verbal instructions may not provide such information.

Points to remember:

1   Graphics are helpful for explaining parallel processes.
2   To aid readers' understanding of risk, use frequencies in both text and graphics.
3   The visual design of tables should show 'at a glance' which items belong together.
4   Design route information to support decision-making both before and during the route.

5.2.4 Graphics can enhance instructions

People sometimes need detailed instructions about how to take their medication or what exercises to do or how to use a product such as an inhaler. There are detailed examples of product instructions in Chapter 3. This section flags three goals you might have when including graphics in instructions: flagging content, helping memory, persuading.

Flagging content
Readers' understanding of instructions can be enhanced by combining graphic styles, adding text to pictures or pictures to text. Adults with relatively low literacy skills had problems taking their medicines at the appropriate times during the day but were greatly assisted by an illustrated medication chart (Kripalani et al., 2007). Many instructions have these twin components of what to do and when to do it. However, people following instructions focus mainly on what actions they have to take, and pay less attention to details about when these actions should be taken. So you may want to use a graphic to flag the importance of waiting until the conditions are right – e.g. taking tablets after a meal. For some healthcare instructions, doing it at the right time may be just as important as doing it at all.

Writing health communication

Helping memory

Writing multi-step instructions as a prose paragraph leaves readers having to chunk the information into steps that can be appropriately carried out, then remembering the correct sequence of steps. The risk is that people try to remember too much, and subsequent forgetting leads to mistakes. The use of graphic sequences to supplement written text can support both the chunking and remembering activities, and these will be considered further in Section 5.3.3.

Persuading

When a health leaflet is instructing readers to modify their life-style (e.g. eat more healthily or have safer sex), graphics can enhance the persuasive impact of the text. The graphics can depict the negative consequences, or later regret, that may follow from ignoring the advice, or the graphics can emphasise the positive consequences that follow from taking the advice. The use of emotional graphics will be briefly touched on below in Section 5.3 in relation to the choice of graphic styles.

When writing instructions:

1 Use graphics to make contingencies salient.
2 Use graphics to help readers chunk the instructions into manageable steps.
3 Use graphics to help people understand both what actions to take and when to take them.
4 Consider using graphics that arouse an emotional response from readers if you are trying to persuade people to change their behaviour.

5.3 Stage 2: selecting among graphic styles

Graphic styles in health information leaflets range from the photographic realism of a skin cancer to abstract diagrams such as family trees and contingency tables. While graphics are often used to represent physical items, they can also help readers understand abstract concepts such as genetic inheritance. Graphics describing the organisational structure of clinic personnel can help patients understand who to contact about what. The two main factors determining which graphic style you choose will always be your audience and the purpose that you want the graphic to serve. Members of your audience may vary in age, gender and literacy (including health literacy). They will also differ in numeracy, social expectations and cultural values. Audience diversity and the multiple purposes you want your graphic to serve means that there will seldom be a 'best' graphic style. So try to identify and exclude the graphic styles that are inappropriate, and then choose freely among those remaining.

Using graphics effectively in text

Here we will consider four graphic styles:

1 small icons;
2 representational graphics (photographs and line drawings);
3 graphic sequences;
4 graphics showing numerical data.

5.3.1 Small icons

There are national and international standards for icons, such as warnings for poisons, but you should bear in mind that the approval of an eminent committee does not guarantee identification and understanding by your audience. Icons can be highly representational, such as an ambulance. They can also be highly abstract, such as the symbol indicating a radiation hazard. The advantage of readers being familiar with an icon may favour representational graphics, but lack of adequate space can undermine this advantage. A detailed representation, even of something as familiar as a clock face, may just puzzle readers if the final size is very small, although at a larger size it may be recognised and understood more rapidly than an abstract shape. This effect of size highlights that design decisions must reflect a confluence of factors, with the result that there is rarely a simple, universal 'best buy'.

As was mentioned in Section 5.1, small icons can be used as markers or flags within a leaflet. They can supplement headings and subheadings, and also be added to running headings in longer documents in ways that help readers rapidly search for a particular section. One example is the use of a child icon within a medication leaflet to draw attention to information that is particularly important in relation to children. The signposting functions of graphics are discussed in greater detail in Chapter 3.

When using small icons:

1 Select small icons that signal either the intended audience or the topic. Check that the icons selected communicate well at the sizes they are being used.
2 Use small icons as flags to show where information relevant to that audience/ topic occurs.

5.3.2 Drawings and photographs

Accuracy

It should not need saying that all illustrations must be factually accurate but in practice this does not always happen. For example, the British Department of Health issued a leaflet showing a dentist wearing a wrist watch and finger ring, and also a dental patient not wearing protective spectacles (Rajal, 2006). Such mistakes can arise from a division of responsibilities between the people generating the graphics and those writing the content, with the final editorial responsibility being unclear. When using graphics you need to check carefully that not only do they communicate the message you want but that they do not include any material that will undermine the reader's confidence and trust in the information.

When to opt for drawings

If you want to depict objects or actions how do you choose between a photographic image and a picture that is purpose drawn? An advantage of drawings over photographs is that they easily allow extraneous information to be omitted. This can make line drawings clearer for some purposes, especially when giving instructions, for example illustrating how a device should be used. Because the omitted information can relate to age, race and gender, line drawings can be more suitable than photographs when texts are intended for a wide audience (see Figure 5.4). Sometimes cartoons can serve similar 'wide audience' functions, for example illustrating exercises to be done.

Line drawings also make it easy to add information to the graphic, perhaps to highlight certain elements or indicate the direction of movement. There is software for achieving similar effects with photographs, but the necessary 'authoring' skills may not be so readily available. A disadvantage of line drawings is that they can appear unreal, technical and difficult. This perceived difficulty is likely to increase if the drawings include graphic elements such as arrows or graphic callouts that expand on some of the details.

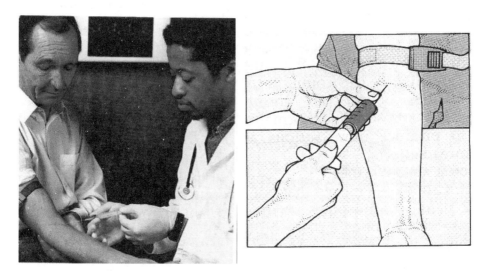

Figure 5.4   Comparison of photographic and line art graphics of an injection. The photograph has more personal impact but the line art has clarity and omits irrelevant details such as age and sex

Source: Tony Smith (2002) *The British Media Association Complete Health Encyclopedia*, p. 276.

Using graphics effectively in text

As has been mentioned, cartoons, i.e. non-realistic drawings, are another graphic style that can be useful, although Hartley (1994) suggests that they probably more often enhance motivation than increase understanding. When sequential or contingent information needs to be given, a cartoon sequence may make the information easier to remember, but care is needed to avoid some readers assuming this graphic style is intended primarily for younger readers, and so ignoring it.

Colour

Another way of changing the appeal of a leaflet can be through colour. The distinction between cognitive and affective consequences can also apply to several uses of colour. A black and white line drawing may adequately convey the information but not add to the appeal of a page in the way that a careful use of colour could. On the other hand, colour can be used to draw the reader's attention to particular items, or it can help to identify features that are discussed in the text. In Figure 5.5 the coloured oval was used to

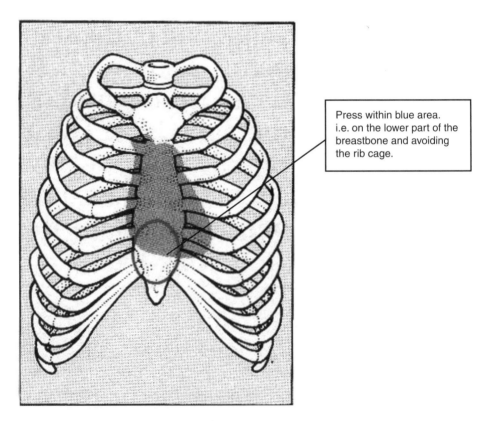

Press within blue area. i.e. on the lower part of the breastbone and avoiding the rib cage.

Figure 5.5 Diagram with a blue oval indicating where to apply pressure during resuscitation (See the colour section at the end of the book)

Writing health communication

emphasise where the hands should be placed when carrying out cardiopulmonary resuscitation.

When to opt for photographs

Among the advantages of photographs, especially those depicting people, is that they can engage readers who will automatically relate to the people shown. To reach a wide audience care must be taken to avoid any unintended narrow focusing that could result from using photographs. One way to do this is to include photographs of a variety of people across an age range and ethnic mix, rather than having the same model patient throughout a leaflet. Variety in the photographs of a medical condition can also be advantageous to those who are trying to help readers identify specific diseases. For example, when explaining how to recognise skin cancers, 'education by photographs' was found more effective than a verbal diagnostic algorithm that relied on a single annotated picture (Girardi et al., 2006). Both for drawings and photographs there can be concerns about the viewpoint from which the graphic is created. A three-quarter view may offer a useful compromise in some contexts, but there will also be instances where showing certain details requires a shift in viewpoint, perhaps to give a close-up or offer separate front and side views. Readers need to be made aware that the perspective has shifted, and not think that the item has enlarged or moved. Figure 5.6 shows how different forms of representation can be combined for this purpose.

Photographs are more likely than line drawings to elicit an emotional reaction from readers. This emotional reaction may be positive (liking) or negative (dislike) which in turn will change people's willingness to read the information at all. Chapter 8 provides a detailed explanation of the considerations and risks of using fear arousing photographs in persuasive messages. As an armchair exercise, how do you think your interest in the eardrum information given in Figure 5.6 would change if the face was ugly?

When using representational graphics:

1 Carefully check the accuracy of all the details in whatever graphics are used.
2 Choose line-drawings rather than photographs for clarity and for audience inclusiveness. Choose photographs rather than line-drawings to heighten the reader's engagement.
3 A variety of photographs can help to offset readers' unintended interpretation of incidental details shown in a photograph, such as age, sex and ethnicity.

5.3.3 Graphic sequences

When using graphics to depict a series of events or actions, you need to adopt a visual sequence that readers will interpret correctly. A single vertical sequence is safe because most people will start at the top and read downwards. Similarly a single horizontal sequence is safe because only a minority of people will try to

Using graphics effectively in text

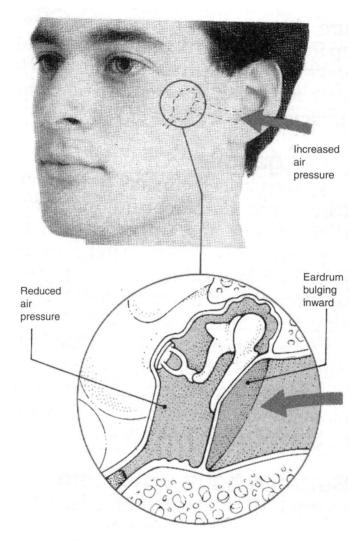

Increased air pressure

Reduced air pressure

Eardrum bulging inward

Figure 5.6   Diagram illustrating how the ears of passengers are affected by the changes in air pressure when planes take off and land

Source: Tony Smith (2000) *The British Medical Association Complete Health Encyclopedia*, p. 159.

read it from right to left rather than from left to right. Other layouts for picture sequences can easily become ambiguous. Arranging pictures in a grid leaves readers uncertain whether they should read down the left column first or across the top row first. Adding numbers to the pictures may resolve this ambiguity, but there can be a risk that these numbers are misinterpreted as indicating something else, such as the frequency with which that action must be carried out. Arrows between the pictures can indicate the reading sequence, but in some contexts may encourage mistaken inferences about causality. The visual sequence chosen should be unambiguous even though this may take more space.

Writing health communication

Add text to graphic sequences

Most readers will have no problems interpreting graphic sequences as being action sequences; nevertheless it is a useful precaution to explain the sequence of actions in words because some people with low literacy skills may not infer the appropriate temporal connections between the pictures, e.g. the need to wait for a tablet to dissolve. When simultaneous actions rather than successive actions are required, such as breathing-in while pressing down on an inhaler, conveying the importance of both actions being done at the same time is best done by adding a text phrase such as '*At the same time*'. There is no reason to assume that graphic sequences must communicate independently of any text (see also Chapter 3). Words and pictures can support each other and sometimes the combination may be essential. The additional text can be integrated with the graphic either by being superimposed on the illustration or given in a figure caption. The crucial point is that the words are not used as a cover for unclear graphics, nor the graphics a means of rescuing unclear text; rather they are being used conjointly to support each other by doing what each does best. That support is greatly weakened if the text and graphics are separated, and it will be unsafe to mention only in the body of the text information essential for the correct interpretation of the graphic because people sometimes read the pictures and the body text quite separately. Action sequences can also be depicted in tables, such as that shown in Table 5.1.

Table 5.1   A table showing how the pattern of taking tablets depends on the age of the person

	Child under 12 yrs	Adult	Senior over 60 yrs
Initial dose (tablets)	1	2	2
Wait (hours)	8	4	8
Another dose (tablets)	1	2	2

When illustrating action sequences:

1 Describe the action sequence in words as well as pictures. Figure captions are often a good way to add verbal information.
2 Add text directly to the graphics where this provides critical information, e.g. '*at the same time*'.
3 Check that graphic sequences are correctly interpreted without people needing to read the body of the text.

5.3.4 Graphics showing numerical data

People have expectations about the meanings of pictorial elements. For example, when graphic elements are arranged vertically, people may ascribe the value 'better' to items depicted as higher. This can pose problems for illustrations such as

Using graphics effectively in text

the food pyramid, which is often incorporated into leaflets giving dietary guidelines. The intended message of the pyramid relates to volume, with foods at the top being those that should be eaten less often; but it is an easy mistake for readers to think that the foods at the top of the pyramid are the Good Foods which should therefore be eaten more often.

Earlier we saw that graphics could help communicate single risks (Figure 5.2), but when people want to compare risks (e.g. breast cancer compared with lung cancer), then simple bar graphs have advantages. Including more than one bar graph in a leaflet may make the information seem too technical for many readers, but if there is good reason to do this then care must be taken that the scales remain constant across graphs, otherwise the message can get distorted. Labelling the bars directly on the graph is more helpful to readers than giving the information in a separate key. As with graphic sequences, if you summarise the intended message of the bar chart in the figure caption this will guide people to focus on the relevant features, and it can reduce misinterpretations. This is also the case with tables. Tables need to have an organising principle that is easy for the reader to spot because this will help them pick out the information that has most relevance for them.

In Table 5.1, the information within a column is visually grouped and the instructions are given vertically because this maps conveniently onto the time sequence once readers have decided which column is relevant. Decisions about what information to put in the rows and what in the columns may sometimes depend on the length of the headings. Longer headings are often easier to accommodate as row headings. It should also be borne in mind that sometimes, especially for instructions rather than explanations, two smaller tables (e.g. for different age groups) may communicate more effectively than one larger but more complicated table. If you decide to include graphics of numerical data:

1   Use data graphics sparingly and in a way that is congruent with readers' assumptions.
2   Be consistent and informative with details such as axes, scales and labelling.
3   Make sure readers can see the organising principle of a numeric table.

5.4 Stage 3: integrating graphics with text

Once you have considered the information needs of your audience, decided on the purposes of your graphics, and chosen the appropriate graphic styles, the final design decision concerns where to locate these graphics within the leaflet. If graphics are serving sign-posting functions, then they will need to be in or adjacent to page margins. In contrast, descriptive and explanatory graphics need to be very close to the text they refer to, and ideally as close to that first textual referent as possible.

Visual proximity is important
When graphics are inserted within a single column of text, readers are more likely to study pictures if they occur immediately after they are mentioned in the text.

Writing health communication

People may be reluctant to stray from the text to a graphic a little distance away, although still on the same page, if they anticipate problems re-locating where they were previously reading in the text. In contrast, if the location of the graphic results in the reader being guided from the text to the graphic and then back to the text, no such problems arise. The value of shepherding readers to the graphic, rather than leaving them to access it when they wish, was also noted in an online study where the graphic was an overview diagram that summarised the links among the characters in the story. This annotated family tree could either be viewed from each page by clicking a button or was shown on the next page as people read through the text. Those people who encountered the graphic as they read had better understanding and retention of the material than those who could access it whenever they wished (Wright et al., 1990). So creating a clear visual path through a leaflet, or providing ways in which readers can go directly to the items of personal interest, becomes one of the hallmarks of good leaflet design.

When the page is divided into two or three columns of text and the graphic spans more than one column, readers may not know where to continue reading even if they ignore the illustration. Do they continue reading in the same column below the graphic or move to the top of the next column above it? There is no consistency in the way magazines, newspapers and web pages make this decision, so even experienced readers can only guess where to continue. *It is best to avoid designs that cause readers to think about the mechanics of reading; readers need to be able to give their full attention to the message.*

In some leaflets even though the flow of the text is linear and no place-keeping problems arise, a graphic is inserted into the middle of the page so that the text flows around it (see Figure 5.7). This disrupts the reading process itself by interfering with normal eye movements during reading. Readers have to hunt for where the text goes next as it flows around the graphic shape. Changing the page layout so that the text maintains the appearance of a conventional paragraph, even though this may mean reducing the size of the graphic, can improve both speed of reading and people's evaluation of how well designed the leaflet is.

Remember when placing graphics in a leaflet:

1 Put graphics close to where they are mentioned in the text.
2 Make it obvious to readers how the text flows around the page.
3 Do not let graphics interfere with the normal, automatic control of reading processes.

5.5 Final note: ensuring that your graphics help not hinder

Among the reasons why leaflets are not always well designed are organisational pressures and conflicting goals, e.g. the tension between taking time to achieve quality versus cutting corners to meet a deadline. The ways in which such conflicts are resolved, and the part that graphics can play in achieving viable compromises,

Using graphics effectively in text

Volunteers wanted

Xxxx xxx xxxxxxxx xx xxxx xxxxxxx x xxx xxxx xxxxxxxx . Xxxxx xx xxx xxxxxx
xx xxxxxxxx x xxxx xx xxxxxxx xx xxx xxxx x xxxx xxxxxxxx. Xxxxxx xx xxxxx x
xxxxx x xxxxxxx xx xxx xxxx xxxxx. Xxxxxxx xxx xx xxxx xxxxxxxx xxx xxxx xx
x xxxxxxxxx. Xxx xxxxxx xxxx xx x xxxxx xxxxx xxx xxxxxx xx xxx xxxxxx, Xx x
xxxxxx xxx xxxxx xxx xx x xxxxxxx.

YYY YYYYYY

Xxxxx x xxxxxxx xx   xxx xxxx xxxxx. Xxxxxxx xxx xx
xxxx xxxxxxxx xxx   xxxx xx x xxxxxxxxx.
Xxx xxxxxx xxxx xx   x xxxxx xxxxx xxx
xxxxxx xx xxx   xxxxxx, Xx x xxxxxx xxx
xxxxx xxx xx x   xxxxxxx.
   Xxxx xxx   xxxxxxxx xx xxxx
xxxxxxx x xxx xxxx   xxxxxxxx . Xxxxx xx xxx
xxxxxx xx xxxxxxxx   x xxxx xx xxxxxxx xx xxx
xxxx x xxxx   xxxxxxx. Xxxxxx xx xxxxx
x xxxxx x xxxxxxx   xx xxx xxxx xxxxx. Xxxxxxx
xxx xx xxxx   xxxxxxxx xxx xxxx xx.

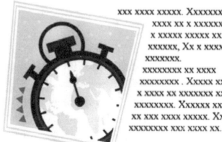

Y YYY YYYYY

Xx xxxxxxxx x xxxx xx xxxxxxx xx xxx xxxx x xxxx xxxxxxxx. Xxxxxx xx xxxxx x
xxxxxx xxx xxxxx xxx xx x xxxxxxx. x xxxxxxxxx. Xxx xxxxxx xxxx xx x xxxxx
xxxxx xxx xxxxxx xx xxx xxxxxx, Xx x xxxx.

YYYYYYYY

Xxx xx x xxxxxxx. Xxxx xxx xxxxxxxx xx xxxx xxxxxxx x xxx xxxx xxxxxxxx .
Xxxxx xx xxx xxxxxx xx xxxxxxxx x xxxx xx xxxxxxx xx xxx xxxx x xxxx
xxxxxxxx. Xxxxxx xx xxxxx x xxxxx x xxxxxxx xx xxx xxxx xxxxx. Xxxxxxx xxx
xx xxxx xxxxxxxx xxx xxxx xx.

YYYYY YYYY YYYY

Xxxxxxx xxx xx xxxx xxxx xxx xxxxxxxx xx xxxx xxxxxxx x xxx xxxx xxxxxxxx .
Xxxxx xx xxx xxxxxx xx xxxxxxxx x xxxx xx xxxxxxx xx xxx xxxx x xxxx
xxxxxxxx. Xxxxxx xx xxxxx x xxxxx x xxxxxxx xx xxx xxxx xxxxx. Xxxxxxx xxx
xx xxxx xxxxxxxx xxx xxxx xx

Figure 5.7   **Eye movement control becomes more demanding when a graphic breaks the flow of the text. Moving the graphic to the side of the page would have been better here**

varies with circumstances and organisations. If you prioritise the needs of your readers, this will increase the chances of your messages getting across to the intended audience. If your leaflet (or notice, or information sheet, or website) fails to communicate, for whatever reason, money is being wasted in producing it at all.

This chapter has emphasised that designers of health information need to consider the purpose(s) of the graphics chosen, their acceptability to the intended audience, plus the graphic options available and their implications for the document as a whole. It will help when juggling all these factors if feedback and advice is received from a range of experts before pilot testing with members of the target audience. Relevant experts include:

- people who know about the specific healthcare domain;
- people who know about the range of graphic design styles that could be used;
- people with editorial skills who can spot ambiguities in graphics and awkward text.

Writing health communication

Different experts will comment on different aspects of the leaflet but no amount of advice will be a substitute for checking that members of the target audience interpret the information as you intend in the context of a leaflet on a specific topic. Advice on how to carry out such testing can be found in Chapters 3 and 4 but see also Dumas and Redish (1999). Heeding the advice from the present book will remove many trouble-spots prior to pilot testing. The list below is adapted from Houts et al. (2006) and will remind you of points covered in this chapter.

Key recommendations:

1 Use pictures to support key points in the text and also to encourage people to read the material.
2 Keep the graphics simple, whether they are drawings or photographs or data charts.
3 Write captions that will help readers focus on the relevant part of the picture and interpret the graphic correctly.
4 Remember graphic representations must be culturally sensitive, and this may be easier to achieve with line drawings than with photographs.
5 When placing graphics on a page, consider both the overall appeal of the layout and the impact on reading processes such as eye movements.
6 Involve health professionals and members of the target audience when creating the graphics. Pictures are not a substitute for unclear language, nor is text a substitute for confusing graphics, but they can be successfully combined to communicate complex information.
7 Graphics can hinder as well as help, so evaluation both before and after publication (e.g. via follow-up interviews) is desirable. This will develop your knowledge of the graphic styles that succeed in your own specialism.

References

Black, A. and Rayner, M. (1992) *Just Read the Label: Understanding Nutrition Information in Numeric, Verbal and Graphic Formats*. London: The Stationery Office.

Dumas, J.S. and Redish, J.C. (1999) *A Practical Guide to Usability Testing* (2nd edn). London: Intellect Books.

Edwards, A., Elwyn, G. and Mulley, A. (2007) 'Explaining risks: turning numerical data into meaningful pictures', *British Medical Journal*, 324: 827–30.

Gigerenzer, G. and Hoffrage, U. (1995) 'How to improve Bayesian reasoning without instruction: frequency formats', *Psychological Review*, 102: 684–704.

Girardi, S., Gaudy, C., Gouvernet, J., Teston, J., Richard, M.A. and Grob, J-J. (2006) 'Superiority of a cognitive education with photographs over ABCD criteria in the education of the general population to the early detection of melanoma: a randomized study', *International Journal of Cancer*, 118: 2276–80.

Griffin, J. and Wright, P. (2008) 'Older readers can be distracted by embellishing graphics in text', *European Journal of Cognitive Psychology*, 21: 740–57.

Hartley, J. (1994) *Designing Instructional Text* (3rd edn). London: Kogan Page.

Houts, P.S., Doak, C.C., Doak, L.G. and Loscalzo, M.J. (2006) 'The role of pictures in improving health communication: a review of research on attention, comprehension, recall and adherence', *Patient Education and Counseling*, 61: 173–90.

Knapp, P., Raynor, D.K. and Berry, D.C. (2004) 'Comparison of two methods of presenting risk information to patients about side effects of medicines', *Quality and Safety in Health Care*, 13: 176–80.

Kosslyn, S.M. (2006) *Graph Design for Eye and Mind*. Oxford: Oxford University Press.

Kripalani, S., Robertson, R., Love-Ghaffari, M.H., Henderson, L.E., Praska, J., Strawder, A., Katz, M. and Jacobson, T.A. (2007) 'Development of an illustrated medication schedule as a low-literacy patient education tool', *Patient Education and Counseling*, 66: 368–77.

Osborne, H. (2006) 'Health literacy: how visuals can help tell the healthcare story', *Journal of Visual Communication in Medicine*, 29: 28–32.

Rajal, A. (2006) 'Poor practice', *British Dental Journal*, 200: 598–9.

Raynor, D.K., Blenkinsopp, A., Knapp, P., Grime, J., Nicolson, D.J., Pollock, K., Dorer, G., Gilbody, S., Dickinson, D., Maule, A.J. and Spoor, P. (2007) 'A systematic review of quantitative and qualitative research on the role and effectiveness of written information available to patients about individual medicines', *Health Technology Assessment*, 11(5): 1–160.

Schriver, K.A. (1997) *Dynamics in Document Design*. New York: John Wiley & Sons Inc.

Springston, J.K. and Champion, V.L. (2004) 'Public relations and cultural aesthetics: designing health brochures', *Public Relations Review*, 30: 483–91.

van Wijk, C. and Arts, A. (2008) 'Does the taxman need a face?' *Information Design Journal*, 16: 85–100.

Wicke, D.M, Lorge, R.E., Coppin, R.J. and Jones, K.P. (1994) 'The effectiveness of waiting room notice boards as a vehicle for health education', *Family Practice*, 11: 292–5.

Wright, P., Hull, A.J. and Black, D. (1990) 'Integrating diagrams and text', *The Technical Writing Teacher*, XVII: 244–54.

Wright, P., Hull, A.J. and Lickorish, A. (1993) 'Navigating in a hospital outpatient's department: the relative merits of maps and wall signs, *Journal of Architectural and Planning Research*, 10: 76–90.

Wright, P., Lickorish, A., Hull, A.J. and Umellen, N. (1995) 'Graphics in written directions: appreciated by readers not by writers', *Applied Cognitive Psychology*, 9: 41–59.

Writing health communication

Developing evidence-based content for health promotion materials

Charles Abraham

In Chapter 4 we explored how the structure of a leaflet, brochure or website directs the way in which readers process information and messages. We noted that it is important to anticipate top-down processes and to structure bottom-up processes. We discussed a series of structural characteristics which help readers use health promotion text efficiently and facilitate intended processing of messages. In this chapter we will consider 'effectiveness' in a different sense. Rather than using design features to enhance processing effectiveness (as discussed in Chapter 4), we will consider the effectiveness of message content in prompting changes in beliefs, attitudes and behaviour. Processing effectiveness facilitates the impact that message content has on individual change but the content of our leaflets and websites is critical to their persuasiveness. In this chapter we will discuss how particular messages target particular cognitive changes by providing information or presenting belief-changing arguments which may in turn change intentions and behaviour.

Learning Outcomes

After reading this chapter, you should be able to:

1 Analyse the message content of health promotion materials, identifying distinct messages and noting the intended effect of each message (e.g., is the message conveying specific information or trying to persuade the reader to adopt a particular belief?).
2 Explain the importance of undertaking elicitation research to discover what needs to be changed in the target audience before designing materials.
3 Consider key theoretical frameworks that specify cognition changes likely to be associated with behaviour change.
4 Assess the extent to which message content addresses cognitions found to be associated with the behaviour being promoted.
5 Assess whether the content of a leaflet or website is well matched to its behaviour change target.
6 Understand the importance of pre-testing health promotion materials to see that they are effective before publication.

6.1 Identifying evidence-based content: research into condom use health promotion

In this chapter we will begin with the example of condom use promotion to prevent sexually transmitted infection, including HIV. First, we will review evidence on modifiable beliefs and attitudes and other such 'cognitions' found to be associated with condom use. Then we will examine leaflets designed to promote condom use and assess the extent to which their content corresponds to research findings on modifiable cognitions associated with condom use. Finally, we will consider an experimental test of an evidence-based health promotion leaflet. Consideration of these studies will illustrate the processes by which research into cognitions associated with target behaviours can facilitate the design of more effective health promotion materials.

In a review of HIV-preventive programmes, Fisher and Fisher (1992) concluded that many were ineffective because the messages they included did not reflect available evidence on the relationship between cognitions (such as beliefs and attitudes) and patterns of behaviour such as condom use. A subsequent review of HIV risk-reduction interventions for adolescents emphasised the importance of this observation (Jemmott and Jemmott, 2000). The reviewers found that interventions that had medium to large effects on cognitions associated with condom use also had significantly greater impact on condom use and on abstinence than interventions that had small or no effects on cognitive antecedents. In other words, when messages targeted how people thought about the target behaviour they were more effective in changing that behaviour. The cognitive antecedents considered in this review were: knowledge about HIV prevention, beliefs about the consequences of condom use for sexual enjoyment, condom use self-efficacy, and HIV preventive intentions. Therefore, ensuring that we can identify relevant cognitive antecedents of a behaviour (or 'cognitions') is foundational to developing texts which will persuade people to change their behaviour. Such research allows designers of health promotion texts to target precisely the cognitions found to predict the target behaviour. For example, if confidence levels in relation to being able to use a condom predicts whether young people acquire and use condoms, then it is important that health promotion texts targeting condom use include instructions on how to acquire and use condoms and emphasise how these tasks can be learnt and managed. For examples of condom promotion interventions which have adopted this evidence-based approach, see Bryan, Aiken and West (1996) and Schaalma and Kok (2006).

6.1.1 Core assumptions underpinning development of effective text-based health promotion

The expectation that leaflets or websites designed to change health-related behaviours, such as condom use, will be effective is based on three assumptions:

Writing health communication

1 We can identify (from research) which cognitions and preparatory actions are associated with the target behaviour.
2 Persuasive messages in health promotion texts directly target these cognitions and actions.
3 Readers are motivated to read and process these persuasive messages.

Yet the design and development of many leaflets are not based on these core assumptions. In this chapter we argue that meeting these assumptions is prerequisite to ensuring the effectiveness of text-based health promotion.

6.1.2 Identifying antecedents of condom use

Publicly available educational leaflets provide information and health promotion relevant to HIV-prevention (including condom use). They can be an important source of health education. For example, a representative survey of young people in Germany found that 50 per cent of respondents indicated they had previously consulted a health education leaflet for information about HIV/AIDS and/or condom use (Bundeszentrale für gesundheitliche Aufklärung, 2004). It is important, therefore, that their potential effectiveness is maximised. Yet evidence regarding the effectiveness of health education leaflets is mixed. Their contents may not be understood, remembered or accepted (e.g., Petty et al., 1993). Moreover, unfortunately, many health education leaflets are not evaluated in terms of their effectiveness.

A meta-analysis is a systematic review of previous studies in a particular area which summarises findings by calculating average effectiveness across studies. A comprehensive meta-analysis summarising evidence relating to social and psychological measures which predict whether or not someone is likely to report using a condom was undertaken by Sheeran, Abraham and Orbell (1999). These reviewers included studies which reported at least one numerical association between a social or psychological measure (including measures of cognitions) and the reported frequency of condom use. The review included data from 129 independent samples. The analyses identified 44 distinct social and psychological correlates. Only seven of these measures met Cohen's (1992) criterion for identifying weighted, average correlations which indicate medium or large effects, that is, associations which indicate an important or useful association with the target behaviour. Consequently, the reviewers identified four cognitions and three preparatory actions which were likely to be useful predictors of subsequent condom use. The cognitive antecedents were: (1) attitudes towards condoms; (2) descriptive norms in relation to condom use (i.e., beliefs that others use condoms); (3) intentions to use condoms; (4) pregnancy motivation (e.g., the belief that condoms can be used as an effective contraceptive as well as protecting from sexually transmitted infections). The three preparatory behaviours were (5) carrying condoms; (6) ensuring condoms were available; and (7) communication with sexual partners about condoms. The reviewers concluded that their results 'provided empirical support for conceptualising condom use in terms of … an extended Theory of Reasoned Action' (Sheeran et al.,

1999, p. 126) and argued that these four cognitions and three preparatory behaviours are important targets for safer sex promotion.

The theories of reasoned action (Fishbein and Ajzen, 1975) and planned behaviour (Ajzen, 2001) have been found to provide useful general guides to cognitions associated with a range of health behaviours. A second meta-analysis (Albarracín et al., 2001) tested the extent to which these two theories were supported by studies of cognitions associated with condom use, and found good support, thereby confirming the findings of Sheeran et al. (1999). Reviews such as these ensure that health promotion designers can meet assumption 1 above, that is, identify cognitions associated with the behaviours they wish to promote. So it is important to read reviews and meta analyses before deciding on the content of persuasive texts.

6.1.3 Are condom-promotion leaflets evidence-based?

Subsequently we examined the content of condom promotion leaflets in two European countries, assessing the extent to which the content of messages included in leaflets was evidence-based (Abraham et al., 2002). A quantitative content analysis (Content Analysis Approach to Theory-Specified Persuasive Educational Communication, CAATSPEC; Abraham, et al., 2007) was employed to categorise messages included in nationally-available leaflets in the UK and Germany. Leaflets included in the study promoted condom use and were widely available to the general population. Thirty-six UK leaflets and 35 German leaflets were identified.

This content analysis research involved development of a coding manual defining 45 types of persuasive message found in the available leaflets. Messages most frequently included were those explaining how people do (or do not) become infected with HIV (6–7 messages per leaflet) followed by messages encouraging contact with healthcare professionals (4–5 in most leaflets). Of the 45 message-types found in the leaflets, only 20 targeted cognitions found to be associated with condom use in previous meta-analyses. Leaflets rightly emphasised the efficacy of condom use, with about three such messages per leaflet with more than 89 per cent of leaflets including at least one such message. In addition, more than two-thirds of leaflets rightly included messages containing instructions on condom use (with 2–4 messages per leaflet).

While this content is encouraging, messages targeting other cognitions found to be associated with condom use were often not included. For example, messages emphasising that others use condoms and approve of partners who use condoms were infrequently included. Similarly, in general, leaflets did not encourage getting condoms, carrying condoms, talking to partners about condom use and the efficacy of condoms as contraceptives. For example, the average number of messages per leaflet for the promotion of getting condoms, carrying condoms and talking to one's partner ranged from 0.03 to 0.64 instances per leaflet. Percentages of leaflets including one instance of each of these three messages were 6 per cent (UK) and 3 per cent (German) for promoting getting condoms, 44 per cent (UK) and 17 per cent (German) for promoting carrying condoms and 17 per cent (UK) and 17 per cent (German) for promoting talking to one's partner about condom use.

The results are illustrated in Figure 6.1. The bars show the size of the association between a particular cognition (i.e., the correlations observed by Sheeran et al., 1999) while the line graph shows the frequency with which UK leaflets included messages targeting that cognitive antecedent. It is clear that the greatest number of messages targeted cognitions less strongly associated with condom use. Cognitions most strongly associated with condom use were often less well targeted – especially messages emphasising the normative acceptance of behaviour such as the belief that others approve of condom use (called subjective norm).

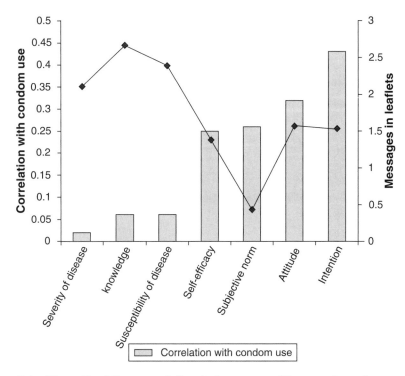

Figure 6.1 **Strength of the association between cognitions and condom use and frequency of messages targeting those cognitions in UK condom-promotion leaflets (Abraham et al., 2002 as reported in Halpern et al., 2004)**

Overall, then, while these nationally-available leaflets informed readers about HIV transmission and warned of the risk of unsafe sex and of the undesirability of STIs, they often failed to include messages that targeted the cognitive antecedents and preparatory actions found to be most strongly associated with condom use by previous research. So while assumption 1 (above) had been met by research, assumption 2 had not been met by the leaflet designers. We concluded that, in general, condom promotion leaflets in the UK and Germany were not evidence-based. We also noted that, while a few significant differences between inclusion of specific message types were observed between UK and German leaflets, the two national samples showed very little cultural distinctiveness in relation to the type of messages they included.

Developing evidence-based content for health promotion materials

6.2 Useful models for identifying and designing the content of health promotion messages

The information motivation behavioural skills model (IMB; Fisher and Fisher, 1992; see Figure 6.2) provides a useful planning tool for thinking about what type of messages are needed in any particular health promotion text. This model implies that the people we want to persuade to adopt beneficial behaviour patterns may need: (1) more information; (2) arguments to bolster their motivation; and/or (3) instruction and explanation to enhance skills needed to perform the target behaviour successfully.

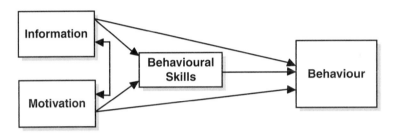

Figure 6.2 The information motivation behavioural skills model (see Fisher and Fisher, 1992)

6.2.1 Elicitation research

The IMB model implies that we need to discover whether our target group lacks any particular behaviour-relevant information, whether key determinants of motivation are in place among this target group and whether the target group lack any skills required to translate motivation into behaviour. For example, if the target audience is well informed but not motivated to change then producing health promotion materials that only provide relevant information will be ineffective. We need to know what cognitive changes are likely to lead to a change in behaviour before we develop health promotion materials. For example, it may be that changing the acceptability of carrying condoms and rehearsing how to use a condom effectively are more likely to promote condom use among a group of young people than providing information about sexually transmitted infections. Consequently, design of effective health promotion texts depends on prior research examining determinants of the target behaviour among the target group and specifying informational, motivational or skill deficits. Such research has been called 'elicitation research' and often involves interviews and surveys with the target group. The results of such research allows health promoters to specify what cognition changes are most likely to promote behaviour change and so allows text design to meet assumption 2 (above).

Findings from the study of condom promotion leaflets described above suggests that health promotion texts are often designed and written on the basis of assumptions about what kind of messages are needed and are most persuasive,

Writing health communication

rather than interpretation of existing evidence or elicitation research. For example, it might be assumed that the risks of not using condoms need to be emphasised, whereas confidence and skills may be the main barriers to condom use among the target audience. If appropriate elicitation research is not conducted prior to the design of heath promotion texts, then these texts may not target the key deficits (in terms of information, motivation and skills) which are preventing the target audience from protecting their health. Thus if health promotion is to be evidence-based and meet assumption 2, it needs to be based on elicitation research.

Of course, sometimes more information is exactly what a target audience needs. In this case elicitation research can identify what kind of information people want. If we do not provide the information people are interested in then they are unlikely to read texts carefully and gain new knowledge. Coulter, Entwistle and Gilbert (1999) reviewed 54 sources of information for patients, including information leaflets. They also conducted elicitation research by listening to patients in focus groups to discover what kind information they wanted. These researchers found that the information included in the sources of information they reviewed did not correspond well to the types of information patients wanted. The researchers generated a list of questions that patients commonly want answered and recommended that patient information sources (such as patient information leaflets) be revised to ensure that they answer these questions (see Box 6.1). Many health promotion texts are not written for patients but the same principle applies. Readers are only likely to be interested in information if it answers questions they are interested in. Knowing what information to provide in a leaflet or website depends on good elicitation research.

Box 6.1 What do patients want to know?

Coulter, Entwistle, and Gilbert (1999) suggest that patients typically want answers to the following questions.

- What is causing the problem?
- Am I alone? How does my experience compare with that of other patients?
- Is there anything I can do myself to ameliorate the problem?
- What is the purpose of the tests and investigations?
- What are the different treatment options?
- What are the benefits of the treatment(s)?
- What are the risks of the treatment(s)?
- Is it essential to have treatment for this problem?
- Will the treatment(s) relieve the symptoms?
- How long will it take to recover?
- What are the possible side effects?
- What effect will the treatment(s) have on my feelings and emotions?
- What effect will the treatment(s) have on my sex life?

(Continued)

Developing evidence-based content for health promotion materials

- How will it affect my risk of disease in the future?
- How can I prepare myself for the treatment?
- What procedures will be followed if I go to hospital?
- When can I go home?
- What do my carers need to know?
- What can I do to speed recovery?
- What are the options for rehabilitation?
- How can I prevent recurrence or future illness?
- Where can I get more information about the problem or treatments?

6.2.2 Targeting Motivation

Unfortunately, even when people have good information, they may not be motivated to change their behaviour. A variety of models and theories have been developed on the basis of previous research to identify key components of motivation. These include the theories of reasoned action and planned behaviour (Ajzen, 2001; Fishbein and Ajzen, 1975). A useful integration of many such theories was undertaken by Fishbein, Triandis, Kanfer, Becker, Middlestadt and Eichler (2001). They identified three prerequisites of action:

1 a strong *intention*;
2 the necessary *skills* to perform the behaviour;
3 an absence of *environmental constraints* that could prevent the behaviour.

These prerequisites correspond to the IMB model in that they specify motivation (that is, intention) and behavioural skills. This framework also emphasises that, sometimes, it is not a lack of information, motivation, or behavioural skills that inhibits action but, rather, the way in which the environment impacts on motivation or the feasibility of action. What is relevant in the environment will vary according to the target behaviour. For example, if people are to be encouraged to wash their hands, then readily-available, attractive hand-washing facilities and fast hand drying options may be critical. So elicitation research also needs to examine environmental prompts and barriers to the target behaviour.

The Fishbein et al. (2001) framework identifies a useful list of cognitions that are likely to enhance and sustain motivation (or intention). These are:

1 The person perceives the advantages (or benefits) of performing the behaviour to outweigh the perceived disadvantages (or costs). This is another way of saying that the person has a positive attitude towards the proposed behaviour.
2 The person perceives the social (normative) pressure to perform the behaviour to be greater than that not to perform the behaviour. This includes

believing that others will approve of their acting in the recommended manner and also believing that other people like oneself are already performing the proposed behaviour.

3   The person believes that the behaviour is consistent with his or her self-image. In other words, they believe that doing what is recommended will make them look good and correspond to how they want to see themselves.

4   The person anticipates the emotional reaction to performing the behaviour to be more positive than negative. So, not only do we want people to believe that the behaviour will be beneficial, but also that they will *feel* good when performing the behaviour or afterwards.

5   The person believes that they can perform the behaviour. This is also referred to as having high self-efficacy. If a person thinks that they lack skills or competence to perform a behaviour, they are unlikely to persist.

The IMB and Fishbein et al. frameworks summarise research into the cognitive antecedents of motivation and action across a wide range of behaviour patterns. They provide a good starting point for thinking about the cognition targets that health promotion is likely to have to change in order to promote behaviour change. Beginning with theoretical frameworks of this kind and then conducting elicitation research is the best way to ensure that health promotion text meets assumption 2 (above).

6.2.3 Targeting self-efficacy and skills

People who believe they can succeed set themselves more challenging goals, exert more effort, use more flexible problem-solving strategies and are more persistent *because* they believe they will eventually succeed. High self-efficacy also helps people focus on a task rather than worrying about their performance and, for example, wondering about personal deficiencies or exaggerating task demands. Such task focus minimises anxiety during performance (Bandura, 1997). Thus self-efficacy boosts motivation and behavioural skills and is a critical prerequisite to effective behaviour change. Bandura (1997) has discussed four main approaches to increasing self-efficacy. First, *mastery experiences* (i.e., experience of successfully performing the behaviour) give people confidence that they can tackle new tasks because they know they have previously succeeded with similar challenges. This recommends that teachers and trainers guide learners towards success by identifying manageable tasks and only increasing task difficulty as confidence and skill grow. The second approach is *observation of others' success*, especially others like ourselves or those we aspire to be like. Thus positive role models (that is, observation of successful others) can enhance self-efficacy. Third, our own *physiological reactions* and our interpretations of these reactions can affect self-efficacy. For example, anxiety during performance can undermine self-efficacy so that interventions designed to reduce anxiety and encourage re-interpretation of arousal (as normal) may facilitate skilled

Developing evidence-based content for health promotion materials performance. Finally, and most importantly here, when direct experience and modelling are not available, self-efficacy can be enhanced through *verbal persuasion*. People can be persuaded by arguments demonstrating that others (like them) are successful in meeting challenges similar to their own (thereby changing descriptive norms), as well as persuasion highlighting the person's own skills, and past success. Therefore, messages in health promotion texts can be designed to increase the self-efficacy of a target audience in relation to a particular behaviour such as carrying or using condoms. For example, a message asserting that, '*Most people need to get used to handling and using condoms but after a little practice people find it easy to use them without interrupting sexual pleasure*', may enhance self-efficacy in relation to condom use by conveying the message that – if most people can do this easily, then so can I. Such a message combined with instructions on how to use a condom correctly and advice to practise condom handling could promote increased self-efficacy and condom-handling skills.

There are many skills that people might need to perfect in order to adopt new behaviour patterns or break existing habits. People can be persuaded to practise such skills by providing self-efficacy-enhancing messages and clear instructions in health promotion texts. New motor skills may be important. For example, in Chapter 2 we saw how health promotion texts can be designed to help people develop the skills to use an inhaler or spacer correctly (see Figure 2.3). Even a simple task like washing our hands to improve infection control may require clear instructions if people are to perform it correctly. Elicitation research can identify the extent to which targeted recipients are proficient or lacking in such skills. Then health promotion texts can be designed to target self-efficacy and skills that are missing in relation to the target behaviour.

Social skills are also often important to behaviour change. Asking others for support and help can often make behaviour change easier. For example, the skills to negotiate condom use with a reluctant partner or the skills to explain why we will not eat traditional but unhealthy foods may be crucial to establishing these health-promoting routines. Identifying who might be helpful to targeted recipients and designing messages that would increase their self-efficacy in relation to asking for help may, therefore, enhance the effectiveness of health promotion texts.

A third group of skills are known as self-regulatory skills. These are cognitive skills which, for example, help people consider longer term consequences of current action, evaluate their current behaviour, set new goals, prioritise goals in the face of other demands, plan action and prompt exertion of appropriate effort when opportunities present themselves. We will discuss the promotion of these skills in more detail in the next chapter. They can be developed using carefully designed health promotion texts. For example, Schinke and Gordon (1992) describe a culturally-specific intervention including a self-completion book using comic strip characters and rap music verse to encourage effective safer sex regulation among black teenagers. The aim was to develop self-monitoring and planning skills as well as verbal resources which can be used to control and disrupt interaction that could lead to unprotected sex. The acronym SODAS, standing for Stop, Options, Decide, Act and Self-praise, was used in this training. The first step, 'stop' focuses on attending to environmental cues and on negative consequences, including emotional consequences, which may follow from failing to plan sexual interaction (e.g., 'stop and think what these choices could really mean for you today, tomorrow … and for years to follow'). Note how this relates to the cognitive antecedents of motivation listed in Fishbein's framework (see cognitive antecedents 1 and 3, above). In this intervention, the text was designed to help the reader think through and plan how they will deal with risky situations. The main aim was not to provide information or change particular beliefs but to develop cognitive resources which will allow the reader to make better future choice. In such cases, texts are being used to develop the readers' self-regulatory skills.

6.3 Matching messages to cognitive targets

Now we would like you to practise targeting messages to particular cognition changes. First, look again at Box 6.1. Any leaflet or website content which answers the questions in this box is providing information; information patients say they want. Next, look at Box 6.2. This box lists a series of persuasive messages that could be used to target key cognitions included in the Fishbein framework – in relation to condom use. Second, think of another behaviour which health promoters might target e.g., increasing exercise or eating fewer calories. (1) Note down messages that provide information that readers might want in relation to the behaviour you have chosen; and (2) list messages that target each of the cognitions included in the Fishbein et al. (2001) framework relevant to the behaviour you have chosen (following the pattern in Box 6.2).

When you have completed these tasks, select a health promotion leaflet (or website) and divide the text into a series of distinct messages. A message may be a complete sentence but a sentence could also include more than one message. For each of these messages decide what kind of change it targets. For example, does it provide information? Does it seek to change normative beliefs? Does it attempt to enhance self-efficacy or teach a self-regulatory skill? When you do this, you will be doing the same type of coding that we did when we coded the content of condom promotion leaflets available in the UK and Germany (Abraham et al., 2002). This exercise is important because it is something we should all do before finalising a persuasive text. We need to clarify exactly what change processes we intend each message to initiate if we are to design effective texts capable of changing readers' cognitions and behaviour. Finally, do you think the leaflet or website you have chosen meets assumptions 1–3 above? If not, how would you improve it?

Developing evidence-based content for health promotion materials

Box 6.2 Messages targeting key cognitions identified by the Fishbein et al. (2001) framework in relation to condom use

Messages promoting the advantages (or benefits) of condom use

- Condoms are effective in protecting against HIV/AIDS.
- Used correctly, condoms prevent pregnancy.
- Using a condom can prolong sexual intercourse.

Messages promoting perception of social pressure to use condoms

- Most young people approve of condom use.
- Most young people who are sexually active carry condoms.
- People who care for you would want you to protect yourself using a condom.

Messages promoting consistency of the behaviour with a positive social image

- Having condoms available and knowing how to use them suggests that you are thoughtful and responsible.
- Being able to use a condom properly shows you are mature and sexually competent.
- Carrying and using condoms is part of being in control of your life.

Messages promoting a more positive than negative emotional reaction

- Using a condom means waking up without worry the next day.
- You can stop worrying and start enjoying yourself when you use a condom.
- You will feel you are caring for yourself and your partner when you use a condom.

Messages promoting confidence or self-efficacy

- It's easy to pick up condoms at your young person's drop in centre. Get some next time you are out.
- Just a little practice will allow you to handle and use condoms quickly. Practise using your fingers.
- Many young people are able to discuss condom use successfully before sex.

6.4 Improving the effectiveness of an evidence-based condom-promotion leaflet

Some leaflets examined by Abraham et al. (2002) met assumption 2. For example, one leaflet included 19 of the 20 messages types targeting cognitions associated with condom use. This leaflet was entitled *Safer Sex ... sicher* (or 'Safer sex... for sure') and published by the German Federal Centre for Health Education (Bundeszentrale für gesundheitliche Aufklärung, BZgA). This leaflet included and repeated messages that: (1) emphasised positive outcomes of condom use (includ-ing protection from STIs and pregnancy prevention); (2) confirmed that others use condoms and approve of their use; (3) instructed the reader on how to use condoms and encouraged him/her to think that they are easy to manage; (4) advised the reader to use condoms during sexual intercourse; (5) provided instruc-tions on carrying condoms and having them available and encouraged readers to think that carrying condoms could be easily managed; and (6) advised readers to talk to sexual partners about condoms and provided instruction on how to do this, as well as encouraging readers that they could manage such negotiations. Thus this leaflet targeted a broad range of cognitions and preparatory behaviours found to predict condom use. Consequently, if readers were persuaded by these messages we would expect them to use condoms more often.

Even when the content of leaflets is well chosen, as in *Safer Sex … sicher*, the effectiveness of the leaflet may be enhanced by motivating readers to pay attention to the messages it includes. Research into persuasive communication, indicates that systematic processing of messages leads to more stable cognitive change than peripheral or superficial processing. Moreover, whether or not people engage in systematic message processing has been shown to depend on their motivation to understand and accept messages (Petty and Cacioppo, 1986). As Petty et al. (1993) note, messages 'will be more successful in producing consequential attitude changes if people are motivated and able to think about the information presented and this processing results in favourable cognitive and affective responses' (p. 175).

Krahé, Abraham, and Scheinberger-Olwig (2005) tested whether an external reward could motivate greater attention to leaflet content and so enhance leaflet effectiveness. They compared teenagers who had read *Safer Sex … sicher* with a similar group who had also read the leaflet but were also invited to complete a quiz asking about the messages it contained. This latter group were told that if they completing the quiz correctly they would be entered into a prize draw and could win attractive music prizes. The idea was to encourage readers to pay atten-tion and to re-read the leaflet in order to prepare themselves for the quiz. This motivational enhancement had the advantage of being practical and sustainable in everyday health promotion practice because BZgA had already established that they could add such a quiz to the *Safer Sex … sicher* leaflet, run occasional prize draws and distribute prizes to people who submitted quiz answers.

Our research question was – would including the quiz and prize draw improve the effectiveness of the leaflet and so result in greater pro-condom cognitive change? Both groups completed the same questionnaire measuring a range of cognitions that had been identified as related to condom use in previous research both before and after reading the leaflet.

Three measures of attitude were included. These were: general attitude towards condom use (e.g., '*Condoms make sex less intimate and romantic*'); attitude towards using condoms with a new partner (e.g., '*Using condoms with a new partner is sen-sible*'); and attitude towards using condoms with a steady partner (e.g., '*Using condoms with a steady partner is pleasant/unpleasant*'). Normative beliefs were also

Developing evidence-based content for health promotion materials

measured. These included normative beliefs with respect to preparatory actions such as carrying condoms (e.g., *'Most boys I know take a condom with them when they go out in the evening'*) and normative beliefs with respect to others' approval of using condoms (e.g., *'Most people who are important to me think I should use a condom every time I have sex'*). Self-efficacy in relation to making condoms available (e.g., *'How easy or difficult would it be for you to make sure to have condoms at home?'*) and in relation to using condoms, was also measured (e.g., *'I am confident I will use a condom every time I have sex with a new partner'*). Other measures included self-efficacy in relation to negotiating condom use with a partner (e.g., *'I would not be embarrassed to suggest to a new sexual partner that we should use a condom'*) and pregnancy motivation (e.g., *'I think condoms are a good method of contraception'*). Motivation was measured by assessing strength of intention (e.g., *'I intend to use a condom every time I have sexual intercourse with a new partner'*).

Results showed that combining the leaflet with a motivational incentive for systematic processing, that is the quiz and prize draw, produced higher average scores on 6 of the 10 measures of cognition (i.e., general attitude, attitude with new partners, attitude with steady partners, self-efficacy for preparatory actions, self-efficacy for condom use and intention). So the leaflet in combination with a motivational incentive for systematic processing generated more cognition change. Thus the enhanced leaflet promoted cognitive antecedents of condom use more effectively than the leaflet alone. This shows that, as well as targeting the content of our texts precisely, we need to consider how readers will use health promotion texts and consider whether we can present them in a manner that makes it more likely that readers will pay attention. If we can enhance readers' attention and motivation to read our texts, it is more likely that they will be persuaded by the messages we have included in our texts. In doing so we can ensure that we also meet assumption 3 (above).

This study can be seen as an example of pre-testing health promotion materials. We noted how important this is in Chapter 2 and we want to emphasise this point again here. By examining what impact a leaflet or website has on a sample of the target audience we may be able to identify problems either with the text structure, the message content or the way the text affects readers' motivation to pay attention. For example, do readers interpret the messages in the same way as designers? Do they find the presentation attractive? Do they want to re-read the text? Identifying the limitations of health promotion materials and developing solutions that improve them before publication is very likely to enhance their effectiveness.

6.5 Conclusion

In this chapter we have focused on ensuring that the messages in health promotion texts (e.g., leaflets or websites) have clear change targets. We have noted that the content of these messages must be matched to cognition changes that are associated with the target behaviour if the text is to be effective.

Writing health communication

We noted that the changes most likely to bring about behaviour change need to be identified using theoretical frameworks based on previous research and by elicitation research. We have considered the Information Motivation and Behavioural Skills model and the Fishbein framework for understanding components of motivation. However, finding out what the target audience already knows, thinks and is able to do through elicitation research is crucial to designing effective persuasive text.

We encourage you to carefully analyse the content of health promotion texts to see exactly what changes messages are targeting. This is a first step towards ensuring that the messages included in a health promotion text are targeting changes most likely to result in behaviour change among the target audience.

Finally, we noted that if readers can be motivated to read health promotion texts carefully and to re-read them, this is likely to result in greater persuasion and cognitive and behavioural change. So ensuring that the presentation of texts holds readers' attention is important. Pre-testing of materials is crucial to ensuring that the message content and the presentation will target important changes effectively. We will take this approach one step further by considering a range of behaviour change techniques in Chapter 7 and, in Chapter 9, we will discuss how this approach can be applied at an individual level, tailoring messages to individualised change targets using computer tailoring.

Note

The work discussed in this chapter was partially supported by the National Institute for Health Research (NIHR) UK. However, the views expressed are those of the author and not necessarily those of the NIHR or the UK Department of Health.

References

Abraham, C., Krahé, B., Dominic, R. and Fritsche, I. (2002) 'Do health promotion messages target cognitive and behavioural correlates of condom use? A content analysis of safer-sex promotion leaflets in two countries', *British Journal of Health Psychology*, 7: 227–46.

Abraham, C., Southby, L., Quandte, S., Krahé, B. and van der Sluijs, W. (2007) 'What's in a leaflet? Identifying research-based persuasive messages in European alcohol-education leaflets', *Psychology and Health*, 22: 31–60.

Ajzen, I. (2001) 'Nature and operation of attitudes', *Annual Review of Psychology*, 52: 27–58.

Albarracín, D., Johnson, B.T., Fishbein, M. and Muellerleile, P.A. (2001) 'Theories of reasoned action and planned behavior as models of condom use: a meta-analysis', *Psychological Bulletin*, 127: 142–61.

Bandura, A. (1997) *Self-efficacy: The Exercise of Control*. New York: Freeman.

Bryan, A.D., Aiken, L.S. and West, S.G. (1996) 'Increasing condom use: evaluation of a theory-based intervention to prevent sexually transmitted diseases in young women', *Health Psychology*, 15(5): 371–82.

Bundeszentrale für gesundheitliche Aufklärung (ed.) (2004) *Aids im öffentlichen Bewusstsein der Bundesrepublik Deutschland 2004*. Köln: BZgA. Retrieved online April 92006: http://www.bzga.de/?uid=c6873bef9ee6938ce07e396559c1771e&id=Seite1417.

Cohen, J. (1992) 'A power primer', *Psychological Bulletin*, 112: 155–9.

Coulter, A., Entwistle, V. and Gilbert, D. (1999) 'Sharing decisions with patients: is the information good enough?' *British Medical Journal*, 318: 318–22.

Fishbein, M. and Ajzen, I. (1975) *Belief, Attitude, Intention and Behavior: An Introduction to Theory and Research*. Reading, MA: Addison-Wesley.

Fishbein. M., Triandis, H.C., Kanfer, F.H., Becker M., Middlestadt, S.E. and Eichler, A. (2001) 'Factors influencing behavior and behavior change', in A. Baum, T.A. Revenson and J.E. Singer (eds), *Handbook of Health Psychology*. Mahwah, NJ: Lawrence Erlbaum Associates, pp. 3–17.

Fisher, J.D. and Fisher, W.A. (1992) 'Changing AIDS-risk behavior', *Psychological Bulletin*, 111: 455–74.

Halpern, D., Bates, C., Beales, G. and Heathfield, A. (on behalf of the Prime Minister's Strategy Unit) (2004) *Personal Responsibility and Changing Behaviour: The State of Knowledge and its Implications for Public Policy*. (www.pm.gov.uk/files/pdf/pr.pdf) London: HMSO.

Jemmott, L.S. and Jemmott, J.B. (2000) 'HIV risk reduction behavioral interventions with heterosexual adolescents', *AIDS*, 14 Suppl. 2, S40–52.

Krahé, B., Abraham, C. and Scheinberger-Olwig, R. (2005) 'Can safer-sex promotion leaflets change cognitive antecedents of condom use? An experimental evaluation', *British Journal of Health Psychology*, 10: 203–20.

Petty, R.E. and Cacioppo, J.T. (1986) 'The elaboration likelihood model of persuasion', in L. Berkowitz (ed.), *Advances in Experimental Social Psychology*. New York: Academic Press, pp. 123–205.

Petty, R.E., Gleicher, F., Blair, W. and Jarvis, G. (1993) 'Persuasion theory and AIDS prevention', in J.B. Pryor and G.D. Reeder (eds), *The Social Psychology of HIV Infection*. Hillsdale, NJ: Lawrence Erlbaum Associates, pp. 155–82.

Schaalma, H. and Kok, G. (2006) 'A school HIV-prevention program in the Netherlands', in L.K. Bartholomew, G.S. Parcel, G. Kok and N.H. Gottlieb (2006) *Planning Health Promotion Programs: An Intervention Mapping Approach*. San Francisco, CA: Jossey-Bass, pp. 511–44.

Schinke, S.P. and Gordon, A.N. (1992) 'Innovative approaches to interpersonal skills training for minority adolescents', in R.J. DiClemente (ed.) *Adolescents and AIDS: A Generation in Jeopardy*. Newbury Park, CA: Sage.

Sheeran, P., Abraham C. and Orbell, S. (1999) 'Psychosocial correlates of heterosexual condom use: a meta-analysis', *Psychological Bulletin*, 125: 90–132.

7

Mapping change mechanisms onto behaviour change techniques: a systematic approach to promoting behaviour change through text

Charles Abraham

In Chapter 6, we saw how the *content of text* can be designed to prompt change in cognitions associated with health-related behaviours. We also saw how integrative theoretical frameworks, which draw upon findings from a wide range of studies, can identify cognition targets, or change mechanisms. Identifying what needs to be changed is a critical first step to developing materials capable of increasing motivation or prompting behaviour change. In this chapter we will develop this idea further so we recommend that you read Chapter 6 before this one.

In this chapter we will discuss health promotion text (for example, in a brochure, leaflet or on a website) as consisting of a series of behaviour change techniques designed to activate particular change mechanisms. We will provide a list of commonly targeted change mechanisms and a menu of behaviour change techniques which can be employed to activate these change mechanisms.

In Box 6.2 we considered how text can be crafted to impact persuasively on five sets of cognitions identified as important components of motivation by the integrative theoretical framework developed by Fishbein et al. (2001). We saw, for example, how messages may be designed to bolster self-efficacy. Enhancing self-efficacy is important to promoting many risk reduction behaviours (see also Chapter 8 on fear arousal, Chapter 9 on framing messages and Chapter 10 on computer-tailored interventions). A series of distinct techniques has been used to enhance self-efficacy (Bandura, 1997). So, the health promoter's task is not just to identify self-efficacy as an important antecedent (or determinant) of health behaviour. The challenge is to identify and implement behaviour change techniques that can effectively promote self-efficacy among the target audience in relation to the target behaviour(s). This is also true of a range of changes that may need to be activated to increase motivation or prompt behaviour change. So, more generally, the challenge for health promoters is to identify and implement behaviour change techniques (BCTs) that can effectively promote the awareness, motivation and skills required to change behaviour. Consequently, effective health promotion requires a mapping of antecedents and determinants, that is the targets we need to change in order to bring about behaviour change, onto a selected set of BCTs that can be used to promote target behaviours among groups where change is needed. Finally, we need to carefully craft text so that it contains the required BCTs.

All behaviour change interventions (including text-based interventions) are composed (implicitly or explicitly) of sequences of BCTs targeting particular change processes or mechanisms relevant to particular behaviours among groups. In this chapter we present a *menu of 40 BCTs* which have been used in previous interventions and from which health promoters can choose when designing text to change motivation and behaviour.

Learning Outcomes

After reading this chapter, you should be able to:

1 Understand the importance of planning to effective intervention design.
2 Consider key elements of the 'intervention mapping' planning process.
3 Building on Chapter 6, identify potentially-modifiable antecedents of motivation and behaviour (including cognitions) which can be selected as change targets when designing text.
4 Select behaviour change techniques likely to activate specific change mechanisms needed to increase motivation or prompt behaviour change.
5 Understand intervention design as a process of identifying and combining appropriate behaviour change techniques.
6 Describe and evaluate approaches to evaluation of behaviour change interventions.

7.1 Planning, elicitation research and mapping change processes onto BCTs

Planning behaviour change interventions involves careful analysis, addressing a series of questions including the following:

1 What is the problem that necessitates intervention?
2 Who needs to change?
3 What behaviours need to be changed?
4 What change mechanisms need to be activated in order to promote changes in awareness, motivation and skills (see IMB – Chapter 6)?
5 What behaviour change techniques can be used to activate these specific changes? How can these behaviour change techniques be written (or built) into health promotion materials?

Writing health communication

Planning is crucial to effectiveness. Peters et al. (2009) conducted a systematic review of reviews examining the effectiveness of school-based health promotion interventions targeting sexual, substance abuse, and nutrition behaviours. These researchers found strong evidence that effective school-based interventions targeting all three behaviours shared five characteristics, namely:

1 the use of theory in intervention design;
2 targeting social influences, especially social norms;
3 targeting cognitive and behavioural skills;
4 training those delivering the intervention;
5 including multiple components in the intervention.

Health promoters need to select appropriate 'theories' that represent the change mechanisms relevant to the problem they seek to address. Not all behaviour change problems will involve changes in norms and behavioural skills (although many will) and not all behaviour change problems require use of multiple behaviour change techniques (although most do). The Peters et al. study does not provide a blueprint for subsequent interventions. Instead, it emphasises that interventions based on careful identification of relevant change processes are more likely to change behaviour successfully.

'Intervention Mapping' (Bartholomew et al., 2011) is a systematic guide to intervention planning. Intervention Mapping highlights six iterative planning stages. These are:

1 needs assessment;
2 matrices;
3 theory-based intervention methods and practical applications;
4 intervention programme;
5 adoption and implementation; and
6 evaluation plan.

We can only briefly consider a few of these stages in this chapter. See Kok et al. (2004) for a brief and accessible introduction to Intervention Mapping and see also the outline planning model presented in Figure 10.1.

Elicitation research (described in Chapter 6) is critical to the 'needs assessment' process. It is essential to know what behaviour needs to be changed. Next it is important to identify underlying change targets and mechanisms likely to lead to behaviour change. This occurs in what is called the 'matrices' stage of Intervention Mapping where potentially modifiable antecedents and determinants (such as cognitions) are identified. The next planning stage is 'theory-based intervention methods and practical applications'. Here, modifiable antecedents are mapped onto behaviour change techniques and these techniques are, in turn, included in materials that allow delivery of the relevant BCTs to the target group. It is this process of translating identified change processes into particular change techniques that we

Mapping change mechanisms onto behaviour change techniques

will discuss in this chapter. We will also return briefly to the important process of 'evaluation' below.

7.2 An intervention planning challenge

The prevalence of people who are classed as overweight or obese is increasing and placing greater demands on health services. Some commercial providers are delivering weight loss classes for local and health authorities. Imagine that we have identified a 'need' to provide an effective local weight loss service and we want to maximise investment by enhancing the weight loss effectiveness of the service offered. How would we do this? Before you read on you might make some brief notes on potential answers to questions 1–6 (above).The problem is already defined. Moving to question 2, perhaps both the people attending weight loss classes and those delivering them need to change. Let's focus initially on the attendees and let's focus on trying to change their dietary and physical activity behaviours (question 3).

Now consider the 11 change mechanisms listed in Table 7.1. Answering question 4, which of these do you think we might need to target to enhance weight loss among people attending local weight loss classes?

Table 7.1   A series of change mechanisms that can boost motivation and prompt action

1. Change beliefs about the benefits and costs of behaviour/s
2. Change risk perception
3. Change feelings (or affective attitudes) associated with adopting or ceasing behaviours
4. Change (normative) beliefs about other people's behaviour and approval of recipients' behaviour
5. Foster a positive behaviour-related identity
6. Enhance self-efficacy
7. Change emotional states in readiness for action and during enactment
8. Prompt and elaborate goals and goal priority
9. Enhance social skills
10. Facilitate behaviour change by prompting environmental change
11. Establish behaviours using rewards

Thinking back to Chapter 6, we can see that – apart from change mechanism 2 (change risk perception), mechanisms 1–6 are those identified by the integrative Fishbein et al. framework as antecedents of motivation. We have also already seen how we might develop targeted text to activate these change mechanisms in written materials (see Figure 6.2).

In this particular challenge, these change mechanisms may not be our priority. We are trying to change people who are already attending local weight loss classes. So, thinking in IMB terms, they are already informed and they are also motivated to change. Consequently, targeting change mechanisms that seek to boost their motivation to lose weight may not be the most effective approach to help them. The exception might be enhancing self-efficacy (change mechanism 6) because people can be motivated and still lack confidence in their abilities. So, in answer to question 4, we might consider change mechanisms 6–11 (in Table 7.1). This is the point at which we need elicitation research. We need to look carefully at the weight loss classes and consider which of these change mechanisms might be most relevant. We might do this by interviewing some of the participants before and after their classes, asking them about how they try to lose weight.

In a real-life version of this challenge, Luszczynska, Sobczyk and Abraham (2007) found that although attendees were setting relevant weight loss goals, their goal setting techniques were not as specific as they could be and were not enabling them to act on their motivation in the right contexts. We, therefore, developed an intervention targeting change mechanism 8 'prompt and elaborate goals and goal priority' (from Table 7.1).

Table 7.2 lists 40 behaviour change techniques used in previous interventions and we can see that four have been used to target change mechanism 8 (BCTs 29–32). Since the attendees were already setting goals, the first of these, BCT 29, was not thought to be useful and so intervention focused primarily on BCT 30 (prompts specific planning) and to some extent BCT 32 (i.e., encouraging people to review and reconsider their previous goals in the light of experience). BCT 30 includes formulation of if–then plans, also referred to as 'implementation intention formation' (Gollwitzer and Sheeran, 2006). Such 'if–then' plans marshal conscious planning processes to cement stimulus-response associations (between the 'if' and the 'then') which later activate behavioral responses. Prompting if–then plans has been found to be effective in isolation and in combination with general action planning across a variety of delivery interventions.

Attendees were taught to make a series of if–then plans specifying precisely when and how they would enact their motivation to reduce calorie intake and increase physical activity. The intervention involved giving attendees planning sheets and teaching them how to use them. The results showed that a one-session intervention added to their classes, based on BCT 30 and 32, could double weight loss (compared to existing classes alone) as assessed by a standard, objective weigh-ins two months later. See Chapter 8 for an effective illustration of how BCT 30 can enhance the effectiveness of fear appeals.

The Luszczynska et al. intervention involved more than just providing written materials. One session of face-to-face tuition was also involved. Nonetheless, it demonstrates how the planning process outlined above can progress from needs assessment (or problem identification) though a series of steps to the selection of specific BCTs and the development of printed intervention materials including those BCTs.

Mapping change mechanisms onto behaviour change techniques

Table 7.2 Behaviour change techniques (that can be incorporated into text) grouped by change mechanisms that can boost motivation and prompt action

Techniques designed to change beliefs about the benefits and costs of behaviour/s – i.e., to change instrumental (or cognitive) attitudes.

1. Provide general information on behaviour–health links

Provide background information about the relationship between behaviour patterns and health. For example, the probably of becoming unhealthy (or remaining healthy) depending on one's behaviour patterns. When this involves a more detailed description of health consequences it overlaps with technique 2 (describe likely material consequences of behaviour).

2. Describe likely material consequences of behaviour

Provide descriptions of what is likely to happen if the person performs a behaviour (or behaviour pattern over time), including the benefits and costs (negative consequences) of action or inaction. This might include descriptions of symptoms, disabilities, or quality of life likely to follow from adoption/cessation of particular behaviour patterns. This may also include benefits that may follow from particular actions (such as reporting symptoms to a doctor). A series of consequences may need to be described. Note while serious consequences may be described, this technique does not necessarily involve emphasising the severity of consequences – see technique 5 (emphasise severity of negative consequences to arouse fear). Moreover, it may be important not to emphasise severity if one wishes to avoid arousing fear.

Techniques designed to change risk perception

3. Emphasise personal susceptibility to negative consequences following from behaviour

This can be achieved by describing the type of person most likely to experience the consequences described using technique 2 (describe likely material consequences of behaviour). When this description matches the majority of people in the target audience – in terms of age, sex or behaviour patterns – it is likely to increase levels of perceived susceptibility among this target group. Personalised statements can also be used addressing recipients directly e.g., 'you are at risk'.

4. Prompt recipients to assess their own risk

Sometimes it is helpful to ask recipients to assess their own susceptibility or risk; asking them to predict what is likely to happen to them if they engage in a particular behaviour. This may help them acknowledge responsibility for the consequences described using technique 2 (describe likely material consequences of behaviour). However, unless this is combined with technique 3 (emphasise personal susceptibility to negative consequences following from behaviour), it may also allow the recipient to rehearse false beliefs about their personal invulnerability.

Techniques designed to change feelings (or affective attitudes) associated with adopting or ceasing behaviours

5. Emphasise severity of negative consequences to arouse fear

Matter-of-fact descriptions of consequences (see technique 2; describe likely material consequences of behaviour) do not necessarily emphasise severity and certainly do not necessarily arouse fear. Graphic depictions or descriptions highlighting death, bodily mutilation or decay, pain or suffering or emotional upset are often used to emphasise the severity of consequences and thereby arouse fear.

6. Describe likely emotional (or affective) consequences of behaviour

This is very like technique 2 (describe likely material consequences of behaviour) but focuses on how a behaviour or behaviour pattern is likely to change how the recipient feels.

Table 7.2   (Continued)

This could involve describing how the person may feel relieved, less worried or elated following adoption of particular health-related behaviours. It may also involve descriptions of negative feelings following risky behaviours. One particular approach that has been tested is inducement of 'anticipated regret' by describing the worry and regret people may feel after engaging in risky behaviours and, thereby, emphasising the benefits of avoiding such strong, negative emotions.

7. Prompt self assessment of affective consequences

Among recipients who have experience of target behaviours, invite recipients to reflect on, describe and evaluate how they felt about performing the behaviour. What did they feel – how good or bad – do they want to feel that way again? This is likely to emphasise the personal relevance of feelings described when using technique 6 (describe likely emotional consequences of behaviour).

8. Induce cognitive dissonance

Cognitive dissonance refers to the discomfort people feel when they are confronted with contradictions in their own thinking. For example, 'I love my children and take care of them' and 'By exposing my children to tobacco smoke I am damaging their lungs'. Being confronted with such contradictions can prompt people to change or evaluate their beliefs and so create motivation to change. They may, for example, re-evaluate their past behaviour and/or formulate a new goal (see also technique 29; prompt goal setting) such as 'I will never expose my children to tobacco smoke again', which removes the discrepancy.

Techniques designed to change (normative) beliefs about other people's behaviour and approval of recipients' behaviour

9. Provide information about others' behaviour

People may hold false beliefs about what others are doing. Informing people about what people are really doing can help people understand that their behaviour is typical or unusual. This information may change recipients' evaluation of their own behaviour. This may be especially useful if the descriptions refer to the group the recipient belongs to (or identifies with) or to people the recipient regards as most important to them (which can be established using elicitation research).

10. Provide information about others' approval of the recipient's behaviour

Information about how people in general or, more usefully, people the recipient values or identifies with, feel about their behaviour can change motivation. Knowing that others will approve – or disapprove – of behaviour can be a powerful motivator because we all need to be accepted by others.

11. Encourage recipients to seek social comparison opportunities

Interacting with others may clarify how they behave and what behaviours they approve of so recipients can be encouraged to involve themselves in groups in which they can compare themselves to others. This may involve encouraging people to join support groups (see also technique 29; prompt goal setting) or to seek out interaction with new people or groups.

Techniques designed foster a positive behaviour-related identity

12. Provide a positive group identity for those engaging in the target behaviour

Social identity is important to all of us so we may be reluctant to adopt or cease behaviours if we see these changes as giving us a less attractive identity. Describing those who already engage in the target behaviour/s in a positive and attractive manner may allow recipients to view the proposed behaviour change as enhancing their identity, thereby increasing their motivation to change.

13. Prompt identification as role model/position advocate

This will involve describing how the recipient may provide a good example to others and affect others' behaviour, for example, providing a good example to children or others in their

(Continued)

Mapping change mechanisms onto behaviour change techniques

Table 7.2   (Continued)

group. By emphasising the leadership and guidance role the recipient can play (for example as a peer educator) this may make the behaviour and associated identity more attractive and so increase motivation to change.

Techniques designed to enhance self-efficacy

14. Use argument to bolster self-efficacy

This involves persuading recipients that they can successfully perform the behaviour, arguing against self doubts and asserting that they can and will succeed. This may include highlighting the success of similar others (see technique 9, provide information about others' behaviour) and/ or emphasising easy aspects of the behaviour which can then be linked to use of techniques 16 and 17 (provide instruction and set graded tasks/goals, respectively).

15. Prompt reattribution of past successes and failures

Past successes may encourage future attempts unless the person explains these successes in terms of others of the environment. These 'attributions' of success away from the person may undermine future motivation. Similarly, explaining past failures in terms of a lack of skill or particular environments may strengthen motivation once skill increases or the environment changes. So, for example, arguing that a recipient can perform a behaviour successfully, despite previous failures, because they can develop new skills or control their environment can enhance self-efficacy and change motivation.

16. Provide instruction

Telling participants *how* to perform a behaviour or the preparatory behaviours needed before they successfully perform a target behaviour can boost self-efficacy for those who lack prerequisite skills. This may involve describing steps and movements and may be enhanced by use of graphics and so be linked to technique 17 (set graded tasks/goals).

17. Set graded tasks/goals

When someone is learning a new skill, beginning with the easy parts, practising them and then learning more difficult or challenging elements, combinations or sequences enhances self-efficacy and skill acquisition. Encouraging recipients to start by setting goals (see technique 29; prompt goal setting) they think are easy, encouraging practice of these initial behaviours (see technique 20; prompt behavioural practice), so enabling recipients to experience success with an element or easy version of the target behaviour, is a good way to initiate skill development and behaviour change. Once initial aspects can be performed successfully then recipients can be encouraged to set more challenging goals to enhance their skills. This may include what may be called prompting generalisation, that is, encouraging recipients to try the established behavioural routine in new contexts.

18. Model/demonstrate the behaviour

Sometimes it is more efficient to show or demonstrate what to do – rather than describe it (as in technique 16; provide instruction). People can often quickly learn what to do through observation. This is easier to do in face-to-face intervention but can also be achieved by use of graphics showing sequences of movements augmented by explanatory text.

19. Prompt mental rehearsal of successful performance

Before practising a behaviour imagining how one will perform it and how one will overcome barriers (see techniques 21; prompt barrier identification and planning in relation to anticipated barriers) can provide useful rehearsal and preparation. So inviting people to imagine performing the target behaviour and what that will feel like (see technique 7) in settings where they will need that behaviour, may further boost their self-efficacy over and above what can be achieved by techniques 14–18, above.

20. Prompt behavioural practice

When people are leaning new skills and behavioural routines, practice consolidates this learning. Advising participants to practice the target behaviour or elements of the target

Table 7.2   (Continued)

behaviour (see technique 17; set graded tasks/goals) in classes or as homework assignments may promote skill development and the consolidation of routines and habits.

21. Prompt barrier identification and planning in relation to anticipated barriers

Inviting recipients to identify obstacles to the target behaviour can enable them to plan new approaches which may ensure success despite barriers. However, it is important to combine these two tasks – identifying barriers alone may reduce self-efficacy! Recipients can be encouraged to think about how they have used their resources and competencies to overcome barriers (similar to those they foresee in relation to the target behaviour) in the past or in other situations. They may also be encouraged to think about new skills they may need to overcome the barriers they anticipate, so returning to technique 17, set graded tasks/goals.

22. Prompt self-monitoring of behaviour

Asking people to keep a record of their behaviour, using a diary or even an objective record (e.g., using an accelerometer such as a pedometer) can clarify how well they are doing, or alternatively, highlight the extent of their risk behaviour this can be a powerful way of increasing self-efficacy and motivation and is especially useful if combined with technique 23, provide feedback on performance.

23. Provide feedback on performance

Providing evaluation of recipients past behaviour is possible in text formats by inviting recipients to complete self assessment exercises which instruct them on how to interpret their scores. Computer tailoring can be used to provide even more powerful personalised feedback over time. Anticipating and receiving feedback may strengthen the effects of self monitoring (technique 22, above).

Techniques designed to change emotional states in readiness for action and during enactment

24. Promote self-affirmation

This involves encouraging people to acknowledge their good and valued characteristics. For example, by writing down one's own desirable characteristics one may feel more positive and accepting of oneself. This can facilitate acceptance of one's susceptibility to risk (see techniques 3–4 above) or acceptance of the negative consequences of one's own actions (see techniques 1–2 and 5–8, above). So when defensive responses (to use of techniques listed above) are anticipated these may be reduced by use of self-affirmation.

25. Promote planned ignoring to change mood or psychological state

Sometimes a key barrier to behaviour change (see technique 21, above) is the person's own psychological state. For example, thinking about the planned behaviour may make the person feel anxious or induce some other negative feelings. Providing instructions on how to self monitor such feelings (see techniques 22 and 7) and then on how to ignore these feeling may facilitate the enactment of goals (see techniques 29 and 30). Recipients may simply be instructed to ignore these negative feelings and focus on acting to achieve their particular goal.

26. Prompt self talk

If recipients face barriers (see technique 21) to enactment of their goals (see techniques 29 and 30) they may be able to bolster their own self-efficacy and motivation during action by means of directed self talk. For example, one can reward oneself after the achievement of a key part of a behavioral routine using self-praise (see technique 40 below) or reaffirm one's self-efficacy. Encouraging recipients to use directed self talk during action (while they develop skills) may facilitate successful enactment of goals. For example, recipients could be encouraged to say to themselves 'Well done [Name] you've done [part X]' or 'I'm going to do this – I know I can', depending on the behavioural routine.

27. Prompt guided imagery to change mood or psychological state

A series of approaches have been developed to help people change their mood including guided imagery. For example, the recipient might be asked to imagine themselves in a very

(Continued)

Mapping change mechanisms onto behaviour change techniques

Table 7.2 (Continued)

safe and comfortable setting in which they feel happy and secure. Then they may be invited to ignore worries and concerns and concentrate of feeling relaxed and confident. This could be used prior to many of the techniques described above, such as technique 19 (prompt mental rehearsal of successful performance).

28. Prompt progressive muscle relaxation.

Instead of using imagery to encourage positive mood and relaxation, recipients may be instructed to use this technique in which they try to tense and then deliberately relax sets of muscles throughout the body. For example they might begin with their toes, move on to their feet, legs, stomach, chest, arms and work towards their neck and face muscles.

Techniques designed to prompt and elaborate goals and goal priority

29. Prompt goal setting

A very basic technique in prompting behaviour change is to invite the recipient to set the goal of changing their behaviour. For example, encouraging the person to make a behavioural resolution (or intention) e.g., 'I will take more exercise next week'. This may be helpful for people who are already motivated and have high self-efficacy, and may be especially useful when delivered by a source with high credibility (e.g., a doctor).

30. Prompt specific planning/goal setting

Encouraging detailed planning of what the person will do makes it more likely that their goal (as set using technique 29, above) is salient in the appropriate situation. This may include a very specific definition of the behaviour e.g., frequency (such as how many times a day/week), intensity (e.g., speed or effort), duration (e.g., how long for) and, importantly, context where it will be performed (e.g., a place or setting or a particular social situation). Specific planning using an 'if–then' format is also called 'implementation intention formation'. For example, instead of 'I will take more exercise next week' (see technique 29 above), resolving that '*if* it is lunchtime, *then* I will take a brisk walk around the perimeter of the park' is more likely to prompt action during lunchtimes.

31. Agree a written behavioural contract

Explicitly writing and/or signing a contract which is given to (or held by) another person may strengthen commitment to a goal by making the recipient accountable to another person who will later provide implicit or explicit feedback (technique 23 above) on the recipient monitored performance (technique 22, above). Consequently, these techniques may be used in combination. Written and signed contracts may be incorporated into computer-tailored interventions and managed by using mail or email follow-up contacts.

32. Prompt review and resetting of behavioural goals

Recipients can be encouraged to review and improve their goal setting after a period of time or after achieving a particular level of success. This may, for example, be a component part of technique 17 (set graded tasks/goals). Re-setting goals may be important to develop greater skill or stamina or because anticipated barriers have prevented the recipient acting on their goals. This technique may be usefully used in conjunction with technique 21 (prompt barrier identification and planning in relation to anticipated barriers).

Techniques designed to enhance social skills

33. Provide instruction on resisting social pressure

Sometimes other people's responses are the main barrier to behaviour change. In this case people may need to develop new social skills before they can successfully implement their behaviour change goals. Instruction (technique 16) is one of a number of techniques that can be used in combination with technique 21 (prompt barrier identification and planning in relation to anticipated barriers) to begin to prepare recipients for social obstacles to change. A variety of approaches have been developed, some of which can be used in text format, including presentation and analysis of dialogue found to be typical of social problems

Table 7.2 (Continued)

among the target group. Video scenarios and live role play with analyses and consideration of alternative outcomes (depending on what an actor does) provide greater opportunities for development of social skills (see negotiation and assertiveness skills training below (34 and 35)).

34. Provide negotiation skills training

Learning to negotiate effectively is a key social skill, foundational to successfully performing and maintaining many behavioural routines that involve others. So providing instruction and explanation which teaches recipients to understand others' perspectives and seek compromises which, for example, empower people with opposing views to create simultaneous gains, may be prerequisite to some forms of behaviour change (e.g., consider condom use). Text formats can provide instruction on how to negotiate about particular behaviours.

35. Provide assertiveness training

Teaching people to honestly express their needs and desires in a non aggressive but confident manner can help them negotiate effectively with others (see technique 34, above). A variety of interactive approaches and skills training classes are available but text formats can provide instruction on how to be assertive about particular behaviours.

Techniques designed to facilitate behaviour change by prompting environmental change.

36. Prompt organisation of social support

Social support can facilitate behaviour change. So recipients can be prompted to seek social support in their environment. For example they may be encouraged to set up their own 'buddy' arrangement where a friend engages in the behaviours with them, or to join existing support groups, or to use negotiation or assertiveness skills (techniques 34 and 35) to remove social barriers to their planned change (see techniques 29 and 30).

37. Teach to use environmental prompts/cues

Often our environment prompts us to undertake motivated behaviours. This is especially true of habitual behavioural routines. For example, we walk into the bathroom before bed and are prompted to brush our teeth. During the development of behavioural routines people can be instructed on how to create and pay attention to environmental prompts. Technique 30 (prompt specific planning/goal setting) may involve making existing cues salient using if–then resolutions. However, recipients can be given or helped to create their own cures in the form of, fridge magnets, written post-its, adhesive dots, etc.

38. Teach to avoid environmental prompts/cues

Existing environmental cues may prompt behaviours and habits contrary to the target behaviour. If these prompts are strong, recipients may be taught to identify and avoid such cues. This has also been referred to as 'stimulus control' and may be combined with a series of techniques such as prompting self talk (technique 26). It may include anticipating social situations likely to reactivate old habits and planning to avoid these situations (see technique 30).

Techniques designed to establish behaviours using rewards

39. Provide contingent rewards

This involves praising or rewarding participants but only when they perform specified behaviours. This overlaps with technique 23 (provide feedback on performance) when praise is offered for successful performance. Other rewards including monetary rewards (such as tokens and vouchers) may be used. This technique can be incorporated in computer-tailored interventions and can be applied to parts of a behavioural routine (see technique 17; set graded tasks/goals).

40. Prompt self reward

If the health promoter cannot provide the rewards (as in technique 39 above) then the recipient can be instructed how to self-regulate by rewarding their own successful performance. Note how this technique may overlap with technique 26 (prompt self talk).

Mapping change mechanisms onto behaviour change techniques

7.3 Beyond single-theory intervention design

Theoretical development is crucial to all sciences because theories identify the mechanisms by which phenomena (including behaviour patterns) endure and change. The integration of different theories is a fundamental challenge for all sciences. This is especially true in the science of behaviour change. Most textbooks dealing with behaviour change list a plethora of theories that purport to identify the most important antecedents or determinants of behaviour change. See Chapter 7 of Abraham, Conner, Jones and O'Conner (2008) for an introduction to theories used by intervention designers in health psychology. The problem is that each of these theories only identifies a subset of the change processes.

Intervention Mapping advises that intervention designers consider a range of relevant theories. This should not be understood as pick-and-mix eclecticism. Rather, combining a careful analysis of the problem with the results of elicitation research, the designer should identify the change processes that need to be activated to bring about the behaviour change relevant to the target group's situation and context. This may necessitate using a combination of theories because single theories may fail to include relevant change processes.

7.3.1 Basing intervention design on a single theory can be problematic if that theory does not include the change processes relevant to your problem

For example, the Fishbein et al. framework (discussed in Chapter 6) encompasses the theory of planned behaviour (Ajzen, 1991), a very successful theory that describes change processes that may be necessary to increase a person's motivation to undertake a specified action. Like other theories of its kind, the theory of planned behaviour makes a valuable contribution to our understanding of key change processes that can be harnessed in intervention design. However, like many other theories, it leaves out many change processes that behaviour change designers need to consider. For example, this theory only considers four of the broad change processes listed in Table 7.1 and would not have provided an appropriate mechanistic basis for the Luszczynska et al. intervention considered above.

7.3.2 It is crucial to consider a range of potentially important change processes when designing behaviour change interventions

The Fishbein et al. and IMB frameworks introduced in Chapter 6 are useful because together they identify a fairly wide range of change processes. However, even the combination of these two integrative frameworks does not cover the range of mechanisms encompassed by the eleven broad change processes in Table 7.1. Moreover Table 7.1 is simply a list of frequently identified change processes. You may wish to extend this list. Until theoretical integration develops further in the behavioural sciences, intervention designers will need to consider a range of change processes, necessitating consideration of multiple theories.

Writing health communication

7.4 From antecedents, determinants and change processes – to behaviour change techniques (BCTs)

Modifiable 'antecedents' or 'determinants' are important because they identify potential 'change processes'. All these terms are used to clarify what needs to be changed to generate behaviour change. They refer to underlying mechanisms by which we can instigate – or activate – changes in our target audience. Identifying these potentially effective changes is crucial to intervention effectiveness. However, identifying the change process we need to target is just the first step towards detailed intervention design. For example, let us return to self-efficacy which is highlighted in many chapters in this book (including Chapters 6, 8, 9 and 10). Research indicates that enhancing self-efficacy – when it is lacking in the target audience – often results in successful behaviour change (Bandura, 1997). Having identified self-efficacy enhancement as an important change process, it is not immediately obvious how we should best achieve this. Table 7.2 lists 10 BCTs that may enhance self-efficacy. Most of these could be incorporated into a health promotion leaflet and all could be included in a computer-tailored intervention (see Chapter 10). The text targeting self-efficacy in Box 6.2 (see the last set of messages) illustrates intervention content based on BCT 14 (i.e. 'use argument to bolster self-efficacy').

A BCT is an approach to bring about a particular, defined change. BCTs themselves need to be clearly defined and distinguished from other BCTs. We have provided definitions of 40 BCTs in Table 7.2. The health promotion materials based on any one BCT may vary, but the change process (or mechanism) they target remains constant (across interventions).

Elicitation research may help us decide which BCT (or combination of BCTs) will be most helpful to our target audience. For example, if an existing class provides good instruction and modelling of target behaviours and we are developing a take-home leaflet to augment such classes, then BCTs 16 (instruction) and 18 (model the behaviour) may not be the best way to enhance self-efficacy for our target group. Alternatively, if attendees find it difficult to follow the sequence of actions being taught (e.g., in a keep fit class), then, alternatively, written materials providing instruction (BCT 16) and modelling the sequences of action (BCT 18) may be ideal. Thus through a process of analysis of the behaviour change problem, elicitation research and consideration of potential change processes and available BCTs we can begin to fine tune our intervention. *We can begin to specify precisely which BCTs we need to incorporate in our intervention materials.*

7.5 Developing and using lists of BCTs

The menu of 40 BCTs provided in Table 7.2 is a collection of commonly used BCTs grouped according to the 11 broad change processes listed in Table 7.1. Again you may wish to add your own BCTs to this list.

Mapping change mechanisms onto behaviour change techniques

A taxonomy of 26 BCTs was reliably identified across a range of behaviour change intervention by Abraham and Michie (2008) who analysed the content of interventions included in three reviews, including interventions designed to promote exercise and healthy eating. The Abraham and Michie taxonomy was extended by Abraham, Kok, Schaalma and Luszczynska (2011) who included a larger number of BCTs linked to specified change processes. Table 7.2 represents a further development of this taxonomy with clearer definitions of BCTs linked to 11 broad change processes. Table 7.2 provides a menu of BCTs which intervention designers can select in constructing interventions.

BCTs 1–13 focus on five broad change processes which research has found to increase motivation. We discussed these in Chapter 6. Intervention designers can ask whether their target audience lacks motivation and, if so, which of these processes (or which combination) might best bolster motivation. For example, do recipients understand the consequences of their current actions and recommended behaviour changes (see change process 1 and BCTs 1 and 2)? If so, then messages like the first set in Box 6.2 could provide a good starting point for developing written messages based on BCT 2. Would messages concerning the way the proposed behaviour change is likely to make recipients *feel* be persuasive (see change process 3 and BCTs 5–8)? If so, then the fourth set of messages in Box 6.2 provides examples of the kind of text needed to implement BCT 6. Elicitation research can help answer such questions.

Note too that Chapter 8 explains how BCT 8 should be used with caution and in combination with BCTs capable of enhancing self-efficacy (14–23). Self-efficacy is crucial to motivation and enactment of intentions. Frightening people who do not feel confident about protecting themselves from threat may not be an effective way to change behaviour.

When recipients are found to have high motivation and high self-efficacy they may still need help with regulating their feelings to allow them to make behaviour changes. In this case, BCTs 24–28 may be useful. In addition, as we saw above, our target audience may benefit from help to set goals and make specific plans to regulate their action in specified contexts. In this case using BCTs 29–32 may be effective.

Sometimes cooperation with others and social support are crucial to behaviour change and BCTs 36–38 focus on how recipients might be empowered to arrange such support. BCTs 36–38 illustrate approaches to environmental change including direct provision of social support. There BCTs may be of less use to designers of health promotion text and, of course, there are many other interventions possible at an environmental level. Finally, BCT 39 refers to the use of rewards to sustain behaviours, especially in the early stages of adoption. BCT 40 can be employed to help recipients manage their own behavioural rewards.

Working through the change processes in Table 7.1 and eliminating those that are irrelevant to the target group can help designers focus on the broad changes they hope to instigate. Then, selecting BCTs from the menu in Table 7.2 allows designers to identify the detailed content of their interventions. Once one or more BCTs have been selected (drawing upon elicitation research)

Writing health communication

designers can begin to craft messages that precisely match the BCT description (as in Box 6.2). In this way their messages are likely to directly prompt changes related to the target behaviour. Characterising the change process that written materials (e.g., the leaflets or website) are designed to activate and precisely identifying the behaviour change techniques that the materials will employ is the best way to ensure that messages are matched to the changes needed by the target audience. This process systematically links the behaviour problem through prerequisite change process to the specific content of messages included in health promotion materials.

7.6 Planning evaluation

Careful planning does not guarantee effectiveness. Despite available advice on design (see Chapters 1–5) and on the selection of content (see Chapters 6–9) designers may fail to capture readers' attention or may select BCTs that are not well matched to the target audience's needs. Consequently, it is important that health promotion materials are evaluated. Evaluation involves research into the following:

1 whether the intervention worked;
2 how well it worked;
3 how it worked;
4 for whom it worked.

Evaluation results can guide new analyses of the problem and new health promotion planning and design. If we know that an intervention – such as a leaflet or website – is not effective, we can begin to discover why it did not work and progress to more effective designs. Without intervention evaluation, health promotion does not advance. This is why the Intervention Mapping process recommends that designers plan evaluation *at the same time* as they plan their intervention.

Evaluation involves comparison of outcomes between those who received the intervention and those who did not. This may involve a no-intervention control group or another intervention group (as is the case when an intervention is compared to existing/routine care) – or both. Typically levels of outcome measures (e.g., time spent exercising or weight loss) in the two groups are compared after one group has received the intervention. We usually expect no difference between intervention and control groups before the intervention is implemented and an improvement in the intervention group (compared to the control group) after exposure to the intervention.

Randomisation of people to the no-intervention control group and the intervention group can control for 'confounding' variables. For example, this could ensure that one group is not already exercising more than the other – which would confound the comparison if we were testing a website designed to promote

Mapping change mechanisms onto behaviour change techniques

exercise. A randomised control trial provides the best indicator of whether an intervention was effective. If a series of randomised control trials have been conducted at different times and in a verity of settings and all show that the intervention is effective then we can safely infer that the intervention is effective and can be used across contexts (see Ioannidis, 2005, for an interesting discussion of the reliability of evaluation data).

The question of how effective an intervention is can be answered by calculating effect sizes. Often d values are used. A d value is simply the difference between the intervention and control group (on a particular outcome measure) divided by the overall variation in scores across both groups. This statistic tells us by how much the intervention group have improved (or not) compared to the control group. Anticipating the likely effect size is important to ensuring that enough people are included in the trial to detect any changes the intervention generates.

Validated measures of behaviour or health are needed to evaluate behaviour change interventions. However, it is also important to measure targeted change processes. For example, did the intervention change risk perception or planning or self-efficacy? Measuring behavioural outcomes and the change processes we targeted can establish whether the intervention worked as we intended. This is referred to as *mediation analysis* and can guide future design. For example, consider a leaflet that successfully activated targeted change processes, such that it successfully enhanced self-efficacy – but *did not* change behaviour. In this case we can conclude that the problem was not the design of the materials themselves – which were successful. Instead, the selection of BCTs undermined effectiveness. It may be, for example, that the leaflet needed to be extended to include new BCTs (other than those targeting self-efficacy) in order to successfully prompt behaviour change.

Interventions may be differentially successful for different groups (e.g., women versus men or older people versus younger people). So it is important to check this during evaluation. This is called *moderation analysis* and is important to future design. For example, a leaflet that is effective in helping women change their behaviour but not men implies that we need to develop a new leaflet for men – so returning to the design questions above.

When an intervention is not effective, it is important to know whether it failed because it was not capable of generating targeted changes (and mediation analyses can help clarify this) or because it was not delivered or used as designed. To answer this question a process evaluation is required. This involves examining the way in which the intervention was delivered or used. We have recommended pre-testing in which designers observe how recipients use written materials as part of the design process. It is also useful to repeat this process during evaluation of the finished product. For example, a leaflet may fail to be effective because the context in which it is read does not allow people enough time to read it. In this case redesigning the leaflet may not be necessary. Instead, the leaflet's effectiveness could be evaluated in a new context because it may be effective when people have more time.

Writing health communication

7.7 Conclusion

This chapter describes a planning process by which designers can link the nature of a behaviour change problem to the exact content of the messages included in written health promotion materials. The process begins by clarifying whose behaviour we are trying to change and exactly what behaviour we are trying to promote. We then recommend that designers consider which change processes are likely to be most important to the target behaviour among the target audience (see Table 7.1). This may be clarified by elicitation research in which we observe the target group and ask them about their beliefs, attitude, intentions and behaviour. Having decided on one or more broad change processes which will be targeted by the materials, we recommend considering a menu of behaviour change techniques that have been used in previous interventions. We defined 40 BCTs grouped according to the change process they target (see Table 7.2). Once a designer has selected one or more behaviour change techniques, the precise form of the messages they need to construct will be much clearer. A key test of messages in health promotion texts is – do they correspond to the behaviour change techniques selected? This can be answered during design by pre-testing the materials. Once the materials are complete they should be evaluated, and we have recommended that this evaluation process focus not only on whether they were effective (or not) but also – how effective were they, for whom and how were they delivered or used in practice? Answers to these questions can guide the development of future materials.

References

Abraham. C., Conner, M., Jones, F. and O'Conner, D. (2008) *Health Psychology*. London: Hodder Education.

Abraham, C., Kok, G., Schaalma, H. and Luszczynska, A. (2011) 'Health promotion', in P.R. Martin, F. Cheung, M. Kyrios, L. Littlefield, L. Knowles, M. Overmier and J.M. Prieto (eds), *The International Association of Applied Psychology Handbook of Applied Psychology*. Oxford: Wiley-Blackwell.

Abraham, C. and Michie, S. (2008) 'A taxonomy of behavior change techniques used in interventions', *Health Psychology*, 27: 379–87.

Ajzen, I. (1991) 'The theory of planned behavior', *Organizational Behavior and Human Decision Processes*, 50: 179–211.

Bandura, A. (1997). *Self-efficacy: The Exercise of Control*. New York Freeman.

Bartholomew, L.K., Parcel, G.S., Kok, G., Gottlieb, N.H. and Fernández, M.E. (2011) *Planning Health Promotion Programs: An Intervention Mapping Approach*. San Francisco, CA: Jossey-Bass.

Fishbein. M., Triandis, H.C., Kanfer, F.H., Becker, M., Middlestadt, S.E. and Eichler, A. (2001) 'Factors influencing behavior and behavior change', in A. Baum, T.A. Revenson and J.E. Singer (eds), *Handbook of Health Psychology*. Mahwah, NJ: Lawrence Erlbaum Associates, pp. 3–17.

Mapping change mechanisms onto behaviour change techniques

Fisher, J.D. and Fisher, W.A. (1992) 'Changing AIDS-risk behavior', *Psychological Bulletin*, 111: 455–74.

Gollwitzer, P.M. and Sheeran, P. (2006) 'Implementation intentions and goal achievement: a meta-analysis of effects and processes', *Advances in Experimental Social Psychology*, 38: 249–68.

Ioannidis, J.P.A. (2005) 'Why most published research findings are false', *PLoS Medicine*, 2(8): e124.

Kok, H., Schaalma, H., Ruiter, R.A.C. and van Empelen, P. (2004) 'Intervention mapping: a protocol for applying health psychology theory to prevention programmes', *Journal of Health Psychology*, 9: 85–98.

Luszczynska, A., Sobczyk, A. and Abraham, C. (2007) 'Planning to lose weight: RCT of an implementation intention prompt to enhance weight reduction among overweight and obese women', *Health Psychology*, 26: 507–12.

Mullen, P.D., Green, L.W. and Persinger, G. (1985) 'Clinical trials of patient education for chronic conditions: a comprehensive meta analysis', *Preventive Medicine*, 14: 75–81.

Peters, L.H.W., Kok, G., Ten Dam, G.T.M., Buijs, G.J. and Paulussen, T.G.W.M. (2009) 'Effective elements of school health promotion across behavioral domains: a systematic review of reviews', *BMC Public Health*, 9: 182, doi:10.1186/1471-2458-9-182.

8

Planning to frighten people? Think again!

Robert A.C. Ruiter and Gerjo Kok

Fear arousal messages, called *fear appeals*, are widely used in health communication. Members of the general population and health promoters who design health communication messages tend to believe in the persuasive power of fear. In this chapter we challenge this belief by examining theory and research evidence relevant to the content, structure and effectiveness of persuasive messages. We will illustrate our argument in relation to the use of health warnings on cigarette packages.

We saw in Chapter 6 that it is important to ensure that the content of health promotion messages is based on relevant, evidence-based theory and elicitation research. Yet research into fear appeals shows that, in most cases, fear appeals are not designed according to our theoretical understanding of how messages can change cognitions and behaviour. Moreover, poorly designed fear appeals can easily result in adverse effects, especially among those who most need to change their behaviour. Our aim in this chapter is persuade you to think twice before deciding to use fear appeals in your health promotion texts. You can judge how effective we have been at the end of the chapter!

We begin by identifying the weaknesses in the use of fear appeals in health communication practice. We will argue that severity information is often the most visible component of fear-inducing health communications, but at the same time, the least persuasive component. We then discuss and illustrate the challenges involved in designing effective fear appeals. These challenges lie in convincing the target audience that the health threat is relevant to their personal lives and in inducing a strong belief in the personal feasibility of the recommended protective action, that is building self-efficacy in relation to that action (see Chapter 6).

We will consider results from laboratory studies and describe alternative change techniques to increase risk awareness (such as message tailoring; see Chapter 10). In addition, we will illustrate how people's confidence in their abilities to perform recommended actions (their self-efficacy) can be increased by using clear action instructions about what to do to avert the threat. Finally, concurring with previous authors in this book (see Chapters 3 and 6), we argue for experimental pre-testing before large-scale implementation to ensure the absence of adverse effects of campaign materials and to test whether text is likely to meet designers' objectives. Knowing about the effects of your health message before large-scale implementation will give you the opportunity to think again before deciding on the use of fear appeals.

Learning Outcomes

After reading this chapter, you should be able to:

1 Make an informed decision about the usefulness of fear appeals in prompting change in your target population.
2 Identify the conditions under which fear appeals may backfire.
3 List the message components that comprise an effective fear appeal and evaluate their relative importance to persuasion.
4 Ensure that messages emphasising perceived susceptibility and severity to a health threat are used in an evidence-based manner.
5 Discuss the pros and cons of using fear appeals.

8.1 Use of fear appeals in current health promotion practice

In 2001, the European Parliament and the Council of the European Union issued Directive 2001/37/EC to put into force the laws, regulations and administrative procedures necessary to ensure that each packet of tobacco products, except for smokeless tobacco products (e.g., chewing tobacco), carry textual *health warnings* emphasising the deathly risks of tobacco use (Fontaine and Engqvist, 2001). In Commission Decision 2003/641/EC of 5 September 2003, the European Commission further extended the directive and urgently advised member states to combine textual health warnings with *graphic warning labels* as, the Commission noted:

> Research and experience in other countries which have adopted health warnings with colour photographs [have] proved, health warnings which include colour photographs or other illustrations can be an effective means of discouraging smoking and informing citizens about the health risks related to smoking. (Byrne, 2003, p. 24)

By providing such advice, the Commission intended to ensure that the content of such health warnings was evidence-based.

To facilitate implementation of the health warnings, the Commission provided a source document with 42 messages for use in each member state. Worldwide, the European initiative is supported by the World Health Organization's Framework Convention on Tobacco Control. Article 11.1.b.V obligates the more than 160 signature countries to implement health warnings on packs of tobacco (WHO, 2009). However, only a few countries have introduced and enforced the use of such images. These include Australia (2006) Canada (2001), Brazil (2002), Singapore (2004), Belgium (2006), India (2007), Romania (2008), the United Kingdom (2008), and Switzerland (2010).

Figure 8.1 provides an example of, respectively, a textual warning issued by the Commission in 2001 and a graphic warning in 2003. The textual warning presents the unequivocal statement that smoking kills in bold type, whilst the graphic message presents an image of decaying lungs. Both of these messages cause an emotional shock reaction and are difficult to ignore.

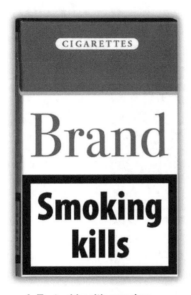 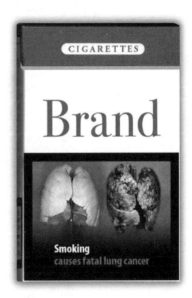

A. Textual health warning   B. Graphic health warning

**Figure 8.1   Examples of fear appeals on cigarette packages in the European Union
(See the colour section at the end of the book)**

© European Union

These warnings on cigarette packages are typical examples of *fear orousing communications*. Similar examples can be found in other health domains. For example, in a New Zealand campaign by Environment Waikato parents were warned of the negative consequences of speeding when driving near schools by a vivid presentation of the bloody consequences which would follow if a child unexpectedly ran into tho road. In a similar way, the Australian government explicitly linked unsafe sexual behaviour with the Grim Reaper (the personification of death) in the mid-1980s to warn people of the fatal consequences of a then new disease called AIDS. Finally, the 'this is your brain in drugs' campaign by Partnership for Drug-Free America (PDFA) used two televised public service announcements (PSAs) and a related poster campaign to illustrate the negative consequences of (excessive) drug use by focusing on the damage done to the brain. Graphic illustrations of these campaigns are shown in Figure 8.2.

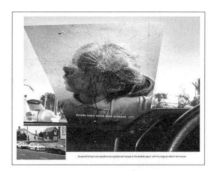
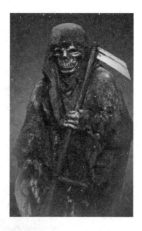
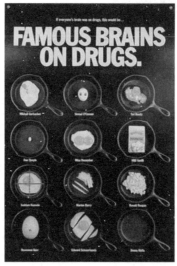

Figure 8.2   Further examples of fear appeal messages (See the colour section at the end of the book)

© Environment Waikato. Available at: http://creativity-online.com/work/environment-waikato-please-dont-speed/8968
© Australian Department of Health. Available at: http://www.avert.org/media-gallery/image-236-the-grim-reaper-australia-aids-campaign-1987
© Capital Concepts, Inc

These campaigns are based on the assumption that by vividly demonstrating negative and life-endangering consequences of risk behaviours people will be motivated to reduce their current risk behaviour and adopt safer alternative behaviours. Is this assumption based on good research evidence?

8.2 Fear appeals are popular

The introduction of health warnings on cigarette packages in 2002 was accompanied by wide-scale media attention on TV, radio and in newspapers throughout

Europe. People in the street, both smokers and non-smokers, were interviewed on their beliefs concerning the effectiveness of these warnings in motivating people to quit smoking. National polls were taken and behavioural scientists were consulted. We ourselves appeared in numerous media items to discuss the use of frightening health messages, especially after the European Commission's decision in 2003 to consider the use of graphic illustrations of the adverse consequences of smoking on tobacco packages.

With the introduction of the 'textual' health warnings in 2002, news items in the media mainly featured supporters of the new warnings, at least in the Netherlands, for example, by reporting on young smokers who stated that they were affected by the message that 'smoking causes ageing of the skin'. Also, soon after the introduction of these messages, national polls were presented that suggested that people smoked less because of the new health warnings. Discussion programmes on radio and television featured people who quit smoking some time after the introduction of the health warnings – while ignoring the fact that many of these people would relapse. Indeed, based on known relapse rates after smoking cessation, as many as 90 per cent of these people may have relapsed (Hajek et al., 2009).

Yet even among those involved in intervention design there is a strong belief in the persuasive efficacy of fear-arousing health messages. A recent meta-analysis (or quantitative literature review) of intervention studies indicated that risk information and information about the (positive/negative) consequences of behaviour are among the two most widely used behaviour change techniques out of 29 techniques identified in a sample of 214 independent research reports (Sheeran, 2006; see also Albarracín et al., 2005).

There is also strong support for the use of fear arousal among politicians and civil servants, bolstered by the advice of the World Health Organization and the European Union to add graphic illustrations to the existing health warnings for tobacco products. It is not clear, however, that this popularity is evidence-based. The evidence used to justify the introduction of graphic health warnings on cigarette packages is apparently to be found in hard-to-obtain governmental reports. Quantitative reviews and peer-reviewed evidence seemed to have played only a limited role in supporting the argument for their use. Moreover, questions could be asked about how available scientific evidence was interpreted.

8.3 Quality of evaluation evidence

Not all evaluation studies provide equally strong evidence of effectiveness. We cannot assume that an intervention which has been supported by research will be effective again (when replicated) unless the evidence produced by the evaluation study is strong. This is why it is wise to consider reviews (including meta-analyses) which summarise the results of many evaluation studies – especially reviews which have selected only evaluation studies reporting strong evidence.

Planning to frighten people? Think again!

Policy-makers may sometimes cherry-pick evaluation studies which support popular policies rather than undertaking a systematic review of available evidence to ascertain the probability of intervention success. Hammond, Fong, McDonald, Brown and Cameron (2004) provide an example of a poorly designed but influential study published in the prestigious *American Journal of Public Health*. The authors concluded that cigarette packet warnings do not have aversive effects and that policy-makers should introduce such warnings without delay. Their evidence is based on self-reports after the introduction of the warnings. Their main argument is that self-reported emotional reactions to the labels predict reported cessation attempts among their respondents at follow-up. This study did not use a control group. Control groups are important because they provide an understanding of naturally occurring change. Therefore, the strength of the presented evidence is weak because the study design does not allow us to draw conclusions about a causal relationship between the introduction of the cigarette warning and reported quit attempts. We cannot assume that the reported quit attempts would not have happened without the introduction of fear-arousing messages. Moreover, the impact of the unmeasured 'third variables' (e.g., price increase, smoking ban) is unknown and the study does not provide us with evidence that quitting percentages after the introduction of warning labels were higher than before (see also Marteau and Hall, 2001; Ruiter and Kok, 2005, 2006). Finally, asking any population of smokers about intentions to quit always results in high percentages of smokers who intend to quit (National Cancer Institute, 2000). Most people who are already smokers want to give up.

Many, apparently effective, interventions cannot be replicated. The strongest research evidence that an effective intervention can be replicated is provided by experimental studies such as randomised controlled trials. A well-designed experimental study allows us to ascertain causal relationships between exposure to the campaign and effects on cognitive antecedents of behaviour (e.g., cognitions such as attitudes and intentions – see Chapter 6) and behaviour (Strahan et al., 2002). An experimental study has a number of key features. Below we have listed features which strengthen the evidence generated by evaluation studies.

1   Inclusion of a control group that has not been exposed to the health promotion message. This group allows us to track what happens naturally without the health promoters' intervention.
2   Ideally participants are randomly allocated to the control group or the experimental group (who receive the health promotion message). Random allocation should ensure that any factors that would change the impact of the campaign are evenly distributed between the control and experimental group. Where random allocation is not possible, researchers try to use matched groups so that the control and experimental groups consist of very similar people who have had similar experiences (Rossi and Freeman, 2004).
3   Use of valid and reliable outcomes measures. These might include previously-tested measures of cognitions associated with a desirable behaviour change, or

Writing health communication

preparatory actions (see Chapter 6), as well as self-reported and objective measures of the behaviour itself. For example, measures of cotinine in saliva can provide an objective measure of whether or not people have smoked recently.

4   These measures are taken from the control and experimental group before and after the experimental group is exposed to the health promotion text. Researchers can then assess differences between the two groups post-exposure and how much each group has changed on each measure.

5   Ideally such studies use large samples which are representative of the target population.

6   Ideally, such studies use long-term follow-up to ascertain whether any observed differences in behaviour are sustained over time.

8.4 Does fear arousal promote behaviour change? Worrying evidence

In experimental social psychology several studies have been reported that tested the effects of frightening health information on persuasion. In contrast to general beliefs about the effectiveness of fear appeals, these studies suggest that fear arousal may easily result in defensive reactions such as risk denial, biased information processing, and allocating less attention to the health promotion messages (e.g., Brown and Locker, 2009). Typically, these defensive responses are most likely to occur among those members of the target population who are most susceptible to the health threat.

One of the first demonstrations of the counter-productive effects of threatening health information was provided by Liberman and Chaiken (1992) who reported that highly relevant information tends to result in defensive processing of the threatening message. They presented coffee-drinking and non-coffee-drinking women with threatening information linking coffee-drinking to the development of fibrocystic disease. The findings showed that women coffee-drinkers, for whom the message was highly relevant, were less persuaded of the link between caffeine and fibrocystic disease than non-coffee drinkers. More importantly, coffee drinkers seemed to have systematically processed the threatening parts of the message, in a defensive, biased manner. Compared with non-coffee drinkers, they were: (1) less critical of information questioning the link between caffeine and fibrocystic disease; and (2) more critical of information supporting this link. In other words, personal relevance may induce defensive processing of health information, resulting in biased processing of threatening information. These results suggest, worryingly, that those most at risk are most likely to reject fear-arousing messages.

In the context of AIDS prevention research, Keller (1999) provided evidence that frightening health messages seem to be least effective for those that are most at risk. Among participants who did not have consistently safe sex during the past six months, that is those for whom the messages were most personally relevant, more frightening messages about the health consequences of unsafe sex (mentioning AIDS-related cancers, syphilis, death) were *less* persuasive and *more* likely to result in message discounting or rejection. Message discounting was shown by greater questioning of: (1) personal susceptibility of contracting sexually transmitted infections (including HIV); (2) the severity of the consequences; and (3) the effectiveness of the recommended action (condom use). In addition, these participants were more likely to reject the message altogether. In contrast, among those participants who consistently used a condom in the past six months, for whom the message would be less personally relevant, those who were exposed to a more frightening message had more positive intentions to use a condom and showed less message discounting than those who received a low fear-arousing message. So fear arousing messages seem to work best for those who least need them!

We have researched whether fear appeals influence the extent to which people attend to health messages. The answer to this question is a definitive yes; we attend to threatening health information, but in a defensive way. Threatening information motivates people to avoid it. In a recent study we recorded brain activity with an electroencephalogram (EEG) and were able to demonstrate that daily smokers attend less to high threatening information about smoking (e.g., picture of a diseased lung) than to low threatening smoking information (e.g., picture of a person holding a cigarette). This effect was not found for non-smokers (Kessels et al., 2010).

Defensive responses to personally-relevant threat information can be understood in terms of cognitive dissonance theory (Festinger, 1957). The theory states that people experience an unpleasant state which they are motivated to change when they become aware of inconsistencies in their belief systems (e.g., I do not want to die. I smoke and smoking will kill me). Dissonance will be reduced if they stop putting themselves at risk by, for example, quitting smoking. However, if this is difficult, as in the case of smoking, an easier way to resolve the dissonance between one's risk behaviour and its negative consequences is by rejecting the message. Biased processing and message derogation can reduce the cognitive and emotional impact of frightening health messages (Keller, 1999; Liberman and Chaiken, 1992) so that the reader may conclude that the threatening message is irrelevant or untrue.

Does fear arousal facilitate behaviour change? No, it does not! At best, it results in maintenance of ongoing behaviour, which is good for people who are not engaging in risk behaviour but bad for people who are engaging in risky behaviour and who are, therefore, the main target audience. The current practice of using fear arousal to motivate at-risk populations to adopt safer behavioural alternatives is at odds with the results of experimental studies. Empirical evidence strongly suggests that people at risk continue with behaviour patterns that have the potential to damage their health when confronted with frightening health messages.

Research suggests that those for whom the threat is most personally relevant are most likely to deny frightening health messages and question their credibility or relevance. Note that personal relevance is usually an important positive feature of health-related messages because it increases attention and cognitive processing

Writing health communication

(see Chapter 10). With frightening messages, this can backfire. Those who most need to change (for whom the frightening message is personally relevant – and personally threatening) are most likely to defensively reject the message.

8.5 What can we do to increase acceptance of fear arousing messages? Encouraging findings

Some research suggests that we may be able to encourage people to attend to threatening health messages, without rejecting them. Although this research is at an early stage, experimental studies suggest that *self-affirming* – a procedure in which people reflect upon cherished values or attributes, for example, responding to questions about their most important values or reflecting on their desirable characteristics – may have the potential to promote more open-minded, balanced appraisal of threatening health messages. For instance, Harris and Napper (2005) found that women who consumed high levels of alcohol but who self-affirmed prior to reading an article about the link between alcohol consumption and breast cancer showed increased message acceptance. These women also saw themselves more at risk, experienced more fear, and exhibited higher intentions to cut down their drinking. In another study, self-affirmed smokers were less resistant to graphic warnings on cigarette packs than non-affirmed smokers (Harris et al., 2007). In the same study, affirmed as opposed to non-affirmed coffee-drinkers were more accepting of the health information used in the Liberman and Chaiken study discussed above. It may be that people are motivated to protect their self-image by denying threatening messages (Sherman and Cohen, 2002). Further research into the potential effectiveness of self affirmation and the promotion of self-efficacy is needed (Good and Abraham, in press).

8.6 Understanding fear appeals

A fear appeal is defined as a persuasive communication that attempts to arouse fear in order to promote precautionary motivation and self-protective action (Rogers and Deckner, 1975). Fear arousal is defined as an unpleasant emotional state triggered by the perception of threatening stimuli. It is assumed that such emotional states involve physiological arousal as well as cognitive, affective and behavioural responses directed towards reduction or elimination of fear.

Fear appeals typically provide two types of information. First, an attempt is made to arouse fear by presenting a threat (e.g., 'cancer') to which the recipient is believed to be susceptible (e.g., 'smoking cigarettes puts you at risk of lung cancer') and which is severe (e.g., 'lung cancer is a deadly disease'). Severity and personal susceptibility information are both necessary to arouse fear. Consider, for example, the case of testicular cancer, which might be a threatening and fear-arousing disease for (young) males, but not for women. Second, a search for 'safety conditions' is prompted by recommending protective action. Acceptance of the recommended action is promoted by presenting the action as effective in neutralising the threat. This is referred to as response-efficacy, e.g., 'by quitting smoking you can prevent lung cancer'. In addition, readers are reassured that the efficacious protective action is easy to execute, that is, readers' self-efficacy is boosted, e.g., 'free smoking cessation groups have been found to help the majority of attendees to give up smoking'. A practical guide for designing effective fear appeals has been designed by Witte, Meyer and Martell (2001).

Several theoretical frameworks have been applied to the study of fear appeals. Protection motivation theory (Rogers, 1983) is the most widely applied scientific model (for a useful overview of this research, see Ruiter et al., 2001). Protection motivation theory suggests that fear appeals instigate two evaluative processes, that is *threat appraisal* and *coping appraisal*. Threat appraisal includes assessments of threat seriousness and personal susceptibility, whereas coping appraisal includes assessments of the effectiveness of potential responses (i.e., response efficacy) and one's ability to undertake these successfully (i.e., self-efficacy). Together these appraisals generate protection motivation or 'the intent to adopt the communicator's recommendation' (Rogers, 1983, p. 158).

The extended parallel process model (EPPM; Witte et al., 2001) develops these ideas and proposes that threat perception initially instigates danger control processes. Danger control is positive because it motivates the reader to take protective, risk-reducing action. So, if the recommended action is seen to be effective and feasible, the person receiving the threat message is likely to follow protective recommendations. However, if coping appraisal suggests that the recommended action is either ineffective or impossible then continuing threat perception will result in ongoing fear arousal. At this point fear control processes become critical in order to reduce the unpleasant feeling. The danger cannot be averted so another way must be found to control fear, for example derogating or denying the threat message. So while danger cannot be averted, the reader can still control and escape fear by message rejection. The EPPM, unlike protection motivation theory, incorporates both danger and fear control processes. Figure 8.3 provides a schematic depiction of the antecedents and consequences of danger control and fear control processes.

Protection motivation theory and the EPPM have been extensively tested and empirical findings have been summarised in several meta-analyses (De Hoog et al., 2007; Floyd et al., 2000; Milne et al., 2000; Witte and Allen, 2000). Experimental and non-experimental studies have found considerable support for the proposed relationships between threat appraisal (i.e., severity, susceptibility), coping appraisal (response efficacy, self-efficacy) and danger control responses, across a wide variety of behavioural domains. In general, perceptions of severity, susceptibility, response efficacy and self-efficacy have been found to correlate positively with measures of protection motivation (i.e., intention to adopt recommended risk-reduction action). However, while associations with risk reduction intentions are relatively strong and consistent for response efficacy and especially for self-efficacy, they are weaker and less consistent for perceived susceptibility and perceived severity (Floyd et al., 2000). In a meta-analysis, De Hoog et al. (2007) found no differences in the effectiveness of messages that used scary images and those that did not. Similarly, in another meta-analysis, Milne et al. (2000) found

Writing health communication

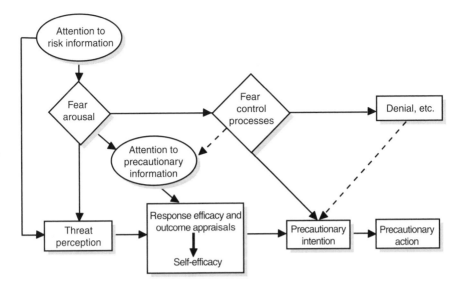

Figure 8.3 Schematic presentation of fear control and danger control processes

Note: Circles represent initial responses to the fear appeal. The diamonds represent automatic emotional responses and are contrasted with conscious cognitive responses that are represented by rectangles. Facilitating effects are represented by continuous lines, the dashed lines represent inhibitory effects.

Source: Ruiter et al. (2001).

that threat appraisal (i.e., severity and susceptibility) and response efficacy measures do not predict future behaviour. By contrast, self-efficacy and intention were found to be strong predictors of future behaviour. Overall, then, the elements of fear appeals most likely to motivate risk reduction behaviours are: promotion of response efficacy (that is, suggesting that the recommended action will avoid the danger); strengthening self-efficacy (that is, suggesting that the person can success-fully perform the recommended protective actions); *not* messages suggesting that the threat is severe or that the reader is susceptible.

In summary, the ideal structure of a fear appeal has changed little over more than 45 years of research.[1] Yet evidence-based theory has not been used to design health promotion messages. Despite the available evidence, designers of frighten-ing health messages continue to emphasise the severity of the health risk in vivid textual and graphic detail. Information targeting perceived effectiveness of the recommended action in reducing the threat (response efficacy), and the per-ceived feasibility of the recommended action (self-efficacy), is often not provided despite being crucial to effectiveness. This poor translation of evidence-based theoretical models explains the counterproductive effects of frightening health messages, especially among those members of the target population who are most at risk. By offering insufficient coping information threatened people feel helpless in dealing with the threat. Denial of the threat is then the only option to avoid the unpleasant feeling that one is at risk of a serious health threat.

Planning to frighten people? Think again!

8.7 Designing evidence-based fear appeals

The main challenge in designing effective health messages concerning health risk behaviour lies in successfully persuading the target audience that they are susceptible to the health threat and, at the same time, inducing a strong belief that they can successfully engage in effective risk reduction actions.

Conveying the message that smoking cigarettes causes serious health problems (severity information) does not necessarily make recipients feel personally engaged with the health problem. Such engagement will depend on acceptance of personal relevance and perceived susceptibility (Ruiter et al., 2001). It is possible for people to acknowledge a threat as relevant (e.g., 'lung cancer is a risk because I smoke') without accepting their own susceptibility (e.g., 'I will not contract lung cancer because neither my mother or grandfather got cancer and both smoked all their lives'). The real challenge is thus in convincing members of the target population that they themselves are at risk, by increasing perceptions of susceptibility. Self-monitoring and feedback can help with this (see Chapter 7). Readers can be asked to self-monitor their own behaviour and then be given a risk assessment based on their own scores. For example, a person can be told (either in person or using computer-tailoring (see Chapter 10)) that they have a low, medium or high risk of disease based on their own behaviour patterns (whether this is smoking, alcohol use, eating, etc.). This process provides personally relevant risk assessments. For example, people with diets that are higher in fat than is recommended by health authorities may believe that their diets are low in fat. Computer-tailoring has been shown to increase susceptibility perceptions, providing an accurate perception of fat intake (e.g., Brug et al.,1998).

We have emphasised the importance of response efficacy and self-efficacy in fear appeals. So, in relation to smoking, we, ideally, want to persuade smokers that quitting will dramatically reduce their chance of contracting lung cancer and that they will be able to quit. Yet smokers are unlikely to succeed without help. When smokers try to quit on their own, 80 per cent relapse within the first week. Only 4 per cent of unaided quit attempts last for 6 months and about 2 per cent succeed permanently (West, 2006; Zhou et al., 2009). When quit attempts are aided by medication and/or behavioural support, 6-month abstinence is observed for up to 9 per cent with minimal intervention strategies (e.g., talking to a family physician) and up to 26 per cent for intensive counselling by a trained counsellor in combination with nicotine replacement therapy (West, 2006).

So instead of emphasising the severity of lung cancer, we should perhaps be advertising the availability of services which effectively support smoking cessation. This was the aim of a UK National Health Service campaign which used the slogan 'Get Unhooked'. This campaign recognised that many smokers want to give up and find it difficult to do so. The images and messages used – such as that in Figure 8.4 – highlighted the difficulty of giving up and emphasised the availability of effective help by giving telephone numbers and websites. This approach is supported by the research discussed above.

Writing health communication

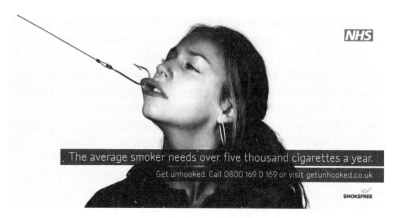

**Figure 8.4   UK National Health Service; Anti Smoking 'Get Unhooked' advert Crown Copyright, Department of Health 2009, available at: http:// smokefree.nhs.uk/resources/resources/product-list/detail. php?code=1724906340
(See the colour section at the end of the book)**

8.8 Bridging the intention–behaviour gap

Besides motivating people successfully to undertake protective action by means of systematically designed persuasive messages, the use of specific action instructions (Leventhal et al., 1965) and volitional prompts (Gollwitzer and Schaal, 1998) can help in bridging what has been called the 'intention–behaviour gap'. This 'gap' arises when people's good intentions to change current risk behaviours are not translated into the effective uptake of less risky behavioural patterns (Webb and Sheeran, 2006).

Leventhal and colleagues studied the relationship between fear arousal and the provision of specific instructions on how to take precautionary action. In one well-known study (Leventhal et al., 1965), participants read a potentially high or low fear-arousing message about the negative consequences of tetanus and were advised to have a vaccination injection at the local hospital. Half the respondents received a map highlighting the location of the hospital and were instructed to think about their daily schedule in order to arrange classes so that they would have time to visit the hospital. This can be seen as an example of combining two behaviour change techniques – a fear appeal and an action planning prompt (see Chapter 7). Results showed that those in the high fear condition had more positive attitudes and intentions towards tetanus injections than those in the low fear conditions. So in this case the fear appeal successfully increased change motivation. By contrast, and unsurprisingly, the provision of planning instructions alone had no influence on attitudes and intentions. Planning instructions did, however, influence action: 30 per cent of the students receiving action instructions had an injection while only 3 per cent did so in the absence of action instructions. Thus fear arousal had a positive effect on motivation but this did not, by itself, result in behaviour change. Motivation was, nonetheless, crucial to action. None

Planning to frighten people? Think again!

of those in the control condition (with no fear message) went for an injection, irrespective of whether or not they received planning instructions. Fear and threat perception created the motivational basis for action while specific planning instructions facilitated the translation of good intentions into action.

These findings foreshadow more recent work suggesting that post-decisional or volitional processes explain why some intenders act while others do not (Abraham et al., 1999). Implementation intentions are a particular form of action planning involving 'if–then' plans, where the 'if' specifies the context or cue in response to which a specified action (the 'then') will be taken. Gollwitzer has argued that such cues prompt intenders to automatically act in accordance with their plan when the environmental cue is encountered (see Gollwitzer and Sheeran, 2006, for a helpful review of relevant evidence). Despite such research evidence, fear-arousing health information is rarely combined with specific action instructions.

Typically we advise people to 'quit smoking now', 'use a condom every time you have sex unless you want to get pregnant', and 'don't drink and drive'. Although most people acknowledge the efficacy of these behavioural recommendations in averting the health threats (response efficacy), they do not help readers to translate precautionary motivation into self-protective action. Clear instructions describing what people need to do are also needed – see Chapter 7. This may necessitate a step-by-step approach in which people start with relatively easy behaviours and gradually move to more complex behaviours (that is, a 'graded steps' approach to behaviour change). For example, the Australian government ran a campaign in which, within the same TV advertisements break, a fear-arousing commercial showing the negative consequences of smoking was then followed by a second television commercial motivating smokers to call the quitline (see http://www.quitnow.info.au/internet/quitnow/publishing.nsf/Content/script-quit). Calling a quit line is an easy to execute action which may provide an effective first step in a successful quit attempt – so this is a realistic behavioural outcome for a mass media campaign.

8.9 Conclusion

We have argued against the use of fear appeals in health promotion practice but emphasised that, if fear arousal is used, it must be used in accordance with research evidence. We have highlighted the weak translation of evidence-based fear appeal theory into the design of threatening health messages. These too often focus primarily on threat severity at the expense of information on how to effectively avert the presented health threat. We have presented evidence showing that information about the severity of possible negative consequences from risk behaviour – the fear-arousing component – is typically the weakest predictor of precautionary motivation and self-protective action. Rather, focusing on severity information is likely to prompt defensive responses. These counterproductive responses may be avoided by providing instruction on how

Writing health communication

to successfully implement the recommended actions as well as convincing people that they are personally susceptible to the threat. So, our advice is to think twice before using fear-arousing messages in your health promotion texts. This book offers many more effective behaviour change techniques – including enhancement of self-efficacy for effective risk reduction actions.

Note

1   The reader may wonder whether the order in which threat information and coping information are presented has an impact on the persuasiveness of fear appeals. No empirical support has been reported for an advantage of the reversed, coping-before-threat format. The threat-before-coping format is the conventional format. This is supported by older (e.g., drive-reduction) and newer theoretical models (e.g., extended parallel process model).

References

Abraham, C., Sheeran, P., Norman, P., Conner, M., De Vries, N. and Otten, W. (1999) 'When good intentions are not enough: modeling postdecisional cognitive correlates of condom use', *Journal of Applied Social Psychology*, 12, 2591–612.

Albarracín, D., Gillette, J.C., Earl, A.N., Glasman, L.R., Durantini, M.R. and Ho, M.H. (2005) 'A test of major assumptions about behavior change: a comprehensive look at the effects of passive and active HIV-prevention interventions since the beginning of the epidemic', *Psychological Bulletin*, 131: 856–97.

Brown, S. and Locker, E. (2009) 'Defensive responses to an emotive anti-alcohol message', *Psychology & Health*, 24: 517–28.

Brug, J., Glanz, K., Van Assema, P., Kok, G. and Van Breukelen, G.J.P. (1998) 'The impact of computer-tailored feedback and iterative feedback on fat, fruit, and vegetable intake', *Health Education and Behavior*, 25: 517–31.

Byrne, D. (2003) 'Commission decision of 5 September 2003 on the use of colour photographs or other illustrations as health warnings on tobacco packages', *Official Journal of the European Communities*, 226: 24–6. Retrieved from EUR-Lex website: http://eur-lex.europa.eu/LexUriServ/LexUriServ.do?uri=OJ:L:2 003:226:0024:0026:EN:PDF

De Hoog, N., Stroebe, W. and De Wit, J.B.F. (2007) 'The impact of vulnerability to and severity of a health risk on processing and acceptance of fear-arousing communications: a meta-analysis', *Review of General Psychology*, 11: 258–85.

Festinger, L. (1957) *A Theory of Cognitive Dissonance*. Stanford, CA: Stanford University Press.

Fishbein, M. and Ajzen, I. (2009) *Predicting and Changing Behavior: The Reasoned Action Approach*. New York: Psychology Press.

Floyd, D.L., Prentice-Dunn, S. and Rogers, R.W. (2000) 'A meta-analysis of research on protection motivation theory', *Journal of Applied Social Psychology*, 30: 407–29.

Fontaine, N. and Engqvist, L. (2001) Directive 2001/37/EC of the European Parliament and of the Council of 5 June 2001 on the approximation of the laws, regulations and administrative provisions of the Member States concerning the manufacture, presentation and sale of tobacco products. *Official Journal of the European Communities* (L 194/26; 18 July).

Gollwitzer, P.M. and Schaal, B. (1998) 'Metacognition in action: the importance of implementation intentions', *Personality and Social Psychology Review*, 2: 124–36.

Gollwitzer, P.M. and Sheeran, P. (2006) 'Implementation intentions and goal achievement: a meta-analysis of effects and processes', *Advances in Experimental Social Psychology*, 38, 69–119.

Good, A. and Abraham, C. (in press) 'Can the effectiveness of health promotion campaigns be improved using self-efficacy and self-affirmation interventions? An analysis of sun protection messages', *Psychology & Health*.

Hajek, P., Stead, L.F., West, R., Jarvis, M. and Lancaster, T. (2009) 'Relapse prevention interventions for smoking cessation', *Cochrane Database of Systematic Reviews* 2009, Issue 1. Art. No.: CD003999. DOI: 10.1002/14651858. CD003999.pub3.

Hammond, D., Fong, G.T., McDonald, P.W., Brown, K.S. and Cameron, R. (2004) 'Graphic Canadian cigarette warnings labels and adverse outcomes: evidence from Canadian smokers', *American Journal of Public Health*, 94: 1442–5.

Harris, P.R., Mayle, K., Mabbott, L. and Napper, L. (2007) 'Self-affirmation reduces smokers' defensiveness to graphic on-pack cigarette warning labels', *Health Psychology*, 26: 437–46.

Harris, P.R. and Napper, L. (2005) 'Self-affirmation and the biased processing of threatening health-risk information', *Personality and Social Psychology Bulletin*, 51: 1250–63.

Keller, P.A. (1999) 'Converting the unconverted: the effect of inclination and opportunity to discount health-related fear appeals', *Journal of Applied Psychology*, 84: 403–15.

Kessels, L.T., Ruiter, R.A.C. and Jansma, B.M. (2010) 'Increased attention but more efficient disengagement: neuroscientific evidence for defensive processing of threatening health information', *Health Psychology*, 29: 346–54.

Leventhal, H., Singer, R. and Jones, S. (1965) 'Effects of fear and specificity of recommendation upon attitudes and behavior', *Journal of Personality and Social Psychology*, 2: 20–9.

Liberman, A. and Chaiken, S. (1992) 'Defensive processing of personally relevant health messages', *Personality and Social Psychology Bulletin*, 18: 669–79.

Marteau, T.M. and Hall, S. (2001) 'EU's anti-smoking stance needs to be more than frightening' (letter to the editor), *British Medical Journal*, 323: 635.

Milne, S., Sheeran, P. and Orbell, S. (2000) 'Prediction and intervention in health-related behavior: a meta-analytic review of protection motivation theory', *Journal of Applied Social Psychology*, 30: 106–43.

National Cancer Institute (2000) 'Population based smoking cessation: proceedings of a conference on what works to influence cessation in the general

Writing health communication

population. *Smoking and Tobacco Control Monograph no. 12*, Bethesda, MD: Department of Health and Human Services, National Institutes of Health, National Cancer Institute, NIH publication no. 00–4892.

Rogers, R.W. (1983) 'Cognitive and physiological processes in fear appeals and attitude change: a revised theory of protection motivation', in J.T. Cacioppo and R.E. Petty (eds), *Social Psychophysiology: A Sourcebook*. New York: Guilford Press, pp. 153–76.

Rogers, R.W. and Deckner, C.W. (1975) 'Effects of fear appeals and physiological arousal upon emotion, attitudes, and cigarette smoking', *Journal of Personality and Social Psychology*, 32: 222–30.

Rossi, P.H. and Freeman, H.E. (2004) *Evaluation: A Systematic Approach* (7th edn). Thousand Oaks, CA: Sage Publications.

Ruiter, R.A.C., Abraham, C. and Kok, G. (2001) 'Scary warnings and rational precautions: a review of the psychology of fear appeals', *Psychology and Health*, 16: 613–30.

Ruiter, R.A.C. and Kok, G. (2005) 'Saying is not (always) doing: cigarette warning labels are useless' (letter to the editor), *European Journal of Public Health*, 15: 329.

Ruiter, R.A.C. and Kok, G. (2006) 'Response to Hammond et al. Showing leads to doing, but doing what? The need for experimental pilot-testing' (letter to the editor), *European Journal of Public Health*, 16: 225.

Sheeran, P. (2006) 'Does changing cognitions cause health behaviour change?' Keynote paper at the 20th Annual Conference of the European Health Psychology Society, September, Warsaw, Poland.

Sherman, D.K. and Cohen, G.L. (2002) 'Accepting threatening information: self-affirmation and the reduction of defensive biases', *Current Directions in Psychological Science*, 11: 119–23.

Strahan, E., White, K., Fong, G.T., Fabrigar, L.R., Zanna, M.P. and Cameron, R. (2002) 'Enhancing the effectiveness of tobacco package warning labels: a social psychological perspective', *Tobacco Control*, 11: 183–90.

Webb, T.L. and Sheeran, P. (2006) 'Does changing behavioral intentions engender behavior change? A meta-analysis of the experimental evidence', *Psychological Bulletin*, 132: 249–68.

West, R. (2006) 'Background smoking cessation rates in England'. Available at: www.smokinginengland.info/Ref/paper2.pdf

Witte, K. and Allen, M. (2000) 'A meta-analysis of fear appeals: implications for effective public health campaigns', *Health Education & Behavior*, 27: 591–615.

Witte, K., Meyer, G. and Martell, D. (2001) *Effective Health Risk Messages: A Step-By-Step Guide*. Thousand Oaks, CA: Sage Publications.

World Health Organization (2009) *WHO Report on the Global Tobacco Epidemic, 2009: Implementing Smoke-Free Environments*. Geneva: World Health Organization. Retrieved from WHO website: http://whqlibdoc.who.int/publications/2009/9789241563918_eng_full.pdf

Zhou, X., Nonnemaker, J., Sherrill, B., Gilsenan, A.W., Coste, F. and West, R. (2009) 'Attempts to quit smoking and relapse: factors associated with success or failure from the ATTEMPT cohort study', *Addictive Behaviors*, 34: 365–73.

Planning to frighten people? Think again!

9

Message framing

Marieke Q. Werrij, Robert A. C. Ruiter, Jonathan van 't Riet and Hein de Vries

To maximise persuasive impact, health-promoting messages usually should contain carefully selected arguments that match specific change targets and include particular behaviour change techniques (see Chapters 6 and 7). This chapter aims at making you aware that it is not only layout and presentation of messages (see Chapters 2–5) and their content (see e.g., Chapters 6–8) but also the precise wording of messages can have an impact on the persuasiveness of the message. This is called 'message framing'.

The following quote appeared on the website of the American Cancer Society (2008):

> Maintaining a healthy weight is important to reduce the risk of cancer and other chronic diseases, such as heart disease and diabetes. Being overweight or obese increases the risk of several cancers, including cancers of the breast (among women past menopause), colon, endometrium, esophagus, kidney, and other organs. Being overweight works in a variety of ways to increase cancer risk. One of the main ways is that excess weight causes the body to produce and circulate more of the hormones estrogen and insulin, which can stimulate cancer growth.

In this example, health risks and negative consequences of being overweight are emphasised in order to motivate people to reduce their weight. This is an example of a 'loss-framed' message: the disadvantages of not performing the healthy behaviour are stressed. If instead, you formulate your message in a 'gain frame' on the other hand, you should emphasise the advantages of performing the healthy behaviour. Thus, the principle of message framing distinguishes two kinds of messages – loss-framed and gain-framed messages:

1   Gain frames emphasise potential gains of your target behaviour, for example, 'If you maintain a healthy weight, you reduce the risk of getting cancer.'
2   Loss frames stress potential losses of not adopting the target behaviour, for example, 'If you are overweight or obese, you increase the risk of getting cancer.'

Note that the message itself is the same in both frames: you want your audience to strive to maintain a healthy weight. Nevertheless, even when the content of messages is kept constant, gain-framed and loss-framed messages have been found to have different persuasive effects.

Thus, to construct effective health messages, it is important to know which frame should be used in order to produce the intended effects. In this chapter we will provide you with clear guidelines about which frame to use in designing effective health messages. However, in some cases, research does not consistently point to a preference for one frame over the other. Which frame is most effective depends on several circumstances. Thus, after a short introduction into the theoretical background of message framing, we will focus on those circumstances under which a gain or a loss frame is more effective.

Learning Outcomes

After reading this chapter, you should be able to:

1 Understand the predictions of prospect theory regarding the different effects of gain- and loss-framed messages on persuasion.
2 Construct gain-framed and loss-framed messages.
3 List factors that may affect when either loss-framed or gain-framed messages will be most effective.
4 Understand the mechanisms behind the effectiveness of gain-framed and loss-framed messages.
5 Choose the most effective message frame when designing campaign materials.

9.1 Message framing and prospect theory

The finding that people respond differently to choices when they are presented in terms of gains or losses is clearly illustrated by an experiment first performed by Tversky and Kahneman (1981). Based on their findings, it was proposed that in general, people are willing to *take* risks when they evaluate outcomes in terms of gains but tend to *avoid* risks when they evaluate outcomes in terms of losses. In this classic experiment called 'The Asian disease problem', people received information about an 'Asian disease' that was about to break out, and that would affect 600 people. Two interventions to combat the disease were presented in terms of gains (programmes A and B) or in terms of losses (programmes C and D). In addition, both the gain-framed messages and the loss-framed messages had one version which was formulated in terms of certain (or definite) outcomes and one version that was formulated in terms of risky (or probable) outcomes. In this way, four different messages were designed. Table 9.1 shows the four messages designed for this experiment.

We can see from Table 9.1 that, in the gain-framed condition, both interventions were presented in terms of the number of lives that would be saved – the gains of the intervention. In the loss-framed condition, both interventions were presented in terms of the number of lives that would be lost – the potential losses

Table 9.1 Four texts used in the 'Asian disease' experiment

	Gain-framed messages	Loss-framed messages
Certain/ definite outcomes	If programme A is adopted, 200 people will be saved.	If programme C is adopted, 400 people will die.
Risky/ probable outcomes	If programme B is adopted, there is a one-third probability that all 600 people will be saved and a two-third probability that nobody will be saved.	If programme D is adopted, there is a one-third probability that nobody will die and a two-third probability that 600 people will die.

Source: Tversky and Kahneman (1981).

Note: Grey boxes indicate the interventions preferred by participants in this study.

of the intervention. In fact, all four programmes have the same expected outcome. The change of wording emphasises gains or losses but does not change the overall outcome. Tversky and Kahneman found in this experiment that when interventions were considered *in terms of gains*, people preferred programme A (the programme with the certain outcome) over programme B. By contrast, when interventions were considered *in terms of losses*, people preferred programme D (the programme with the risky outcome) over programme C – as highlighted by the grey boxes in Table 9.1. Based on these findings, it was proposed that, in general, people are willing to take risks when they evaluate outcomes in terms of costs, or losses, but tend to avoid risks when they evaluate outcomes in terms of gains (prospect theory: Tversky and Kahneman, 1981).

9.2 Perceived 'riskiness' of health-related behaviours

The implication for practice is that health promoters need to know whether their readers view the outcomes of a target behaviour as 'risky' or not. The theory predicts that if they see the target behaviour as risky, they are motivated best by loss frames. If the target behaviour is seen as 'safe', gain frames are the recommended strategy.

So what is a 'risky' health-related behaviour? Preventive behaviours such as sunscreen use and exercising are undertaken to maintain one's health and so tend to be perceived as relatively safe, entailing low risk. By contrast, detection behaviours such as breast or testicular self-examination are thought to be highly risky because, despite the potential long-term benefits, there is an immediate risk of discovering a worrying problem. It has been predicted, therefore, that health promotion messages about (relatively safe) preventive behaviours will be most effective when they focus upon potential gains following the behaviour, while messages about (relatively risky) detection behaviours will be most effective when they focus upon potential losses or costs of not performing the recommended action (Rothman and Salovey, 1997).

These predictions have been supported by a number of studies. For example, Detweiler, Bedell, Salovey, Pronin, and Rothman (1999) gave people going to the beach messages which either emphasised gains associated with sunscreen use (e.g., 'If you use sunscreen with SPF 15 or higher, you increase your chances of keeping your skin healthy and your life long'), or losses associated with not using sunscreen (e.g., 'If you don't use sunscreen with SPF 15 or higher, you decrease your chances of keeping your skin healthy and your life long'). They found that those who read the gain-focused messages were more likely to redeem a coupon to collect sunscreen. Moreover, this (gain-focused) group were more likely to intend to use sunscreen with a sun protection factor of 15 and to intend to apply sunscreen repeatedly. So, in this study, the applied predictions following from prospect theory were supported: a low-risk preventive behaviour was most effectively promoted by gain-framed messages.

Several authors, however, have argued against the proposal that gain-framed messages are more persuasive for prevention behaviours and loss-framed information is more persuasive for detection behaviours. For instance, the assumption that detection behaviours are generally perceived as more risky is questionable. Although people may perceive detection behaviours as having potentially unfavourable outcomes in the short run, it is less clear why people should perceive detection behaviour as dangerous in the long run (Cox et al., 2006). In addition to these theoretical objections, a statistical re-analysis of 53 empirical studies found only a small advantage for loss frames over gain frames for messages advocating breast cancer detection behaviours, but not for any other kind of detection behaviour (detection of skin cancer, other cancers, dental problems, or miscellaneous other diseases). Also, a similar analysis of 93 studies focusing on the predicted advantage of gain frames over loss frames for prevention behaviours only found support for an advantage of gain frames in a limited set of studies, which targeted dental hygiene behaviours. For other preventive health behaviours (i.e., safe sex, sunscreen use, healthy diet), no clear advantage was found for gain frames over loss frames (O'Keefe and Jensen, 2007, 2009).

Thus, the simple version of prospect theory that focused only on the purpose of health-related behaviour (detection or prevention of disease) cannot be used to base your choice on for a gain or loss frame; things are more complicated.

Researchers have searched for other mechanisms that could explain the effects of message framing. Knowing these mechanisms could help health promotion designers assess the specific circumstances their target audience are in, and based on that, they can decide for a gain or loss frame to reach their audience.

Three such mechanisms have been found to influence the effects of message frames and thus may make a difference in your choice for either gain or loss frames:

1 the perceived 'riskiness' of health behaviours by your audience;
2 the expected feasibility of the recommended health behaviour (i.e., self-efficacy);
3 the extent to which a 'fit' is established between the message frame and the receiver.

We will explain each in turn.

9.3 Re-evaluating the concept of 'risk perception'

One reason for the lack of support for the above reasoning with regard to the purpose of health behaviour (prevention vs. detection) is that not all preventive behaviours are perceived as low in risk and not all detection behaviours are perceived as high in risk.

Consider parents' decisions to have their children vaccinated against measles, mumps and rubella using the combined MMR injection. This is a preventive behaviour and so might be assumed to entail low risk. However, publication of – now refuted – reports linking MMR vaccination with autism and inflammatory bowel disease may have changed parents' perceptions of this vaccine. It is possible that they now regard MMR vaccination as a 'risky' behaviour. If this is the case, then according to prospect theory, vaccination would be most effectively prompted, not by focusing on gains, but rather on the potential losses of not vaccinating your child. This was tested and confirmed by Abhyankar, O'Connor and Lawton (2008). They found that a loss-framed message was more effective in increasing women's intentions to have their children vaccinated, than a gain-framed message. Specifically, the loss-framed message: 'By not vaccinating your child against mumps, measles and rubella, you will fail to protect your child against contracting these diseases', was more effective than the gain-framed version of the same message: 'By vaccinating your child against mumps, measles and rubella, you will be able to protect your child against contracting these diseases.'

Thus, your audience's own perception of the riskiness of certain health behaviours is crucial. This was also supported by Apanovitch, McCarthy and Salovey (2003). These researchers found that women who felt safe about the outcome of a HIV-test because they considered themselves not to be at risk, were more likely to report having the test six months after watching a gain-framed video message than those who had seen a loss-framed video message.

The implication of these findings for health promoters is that we cannot assume which behaviours are risky and which are not. You need to understand how risky a recommended health behaviour is in the eyes of your target audience before deciding to design gain-framed or loss-framed messages.

To find out your target audience's perceptions of how 'risky' the behaviour you recommend is, you should use elicitation research (see Chapter 6). For example, when designing a walking intervention for individual post-stroke patients and the intervention is entirely personalised, you should first find out at the individual level whether walking is considered by the patient as involving certain risks (e.g., falling, traffic safety) or if the patient mainly sees advantages of walking (e.g., becoming fit again, enjoying nature). With this information you can effectively use message framing to further enhance the persuasiveness of your intervention. *The advice is then to use a loss-frame if performing the behaviour is perceived to be risky by the target audience, and a gain frame if performance of the behaviour is believed to entail low risk.*

If elicitation research is not possible and you are thus unsure about the perceived riskiness of the behaviour, we advise you to use a gain frame. The reason is

Writing health communication

that loss-framed messages are inherently risky by themselves. That is, loss-framed messages have been found to evoke a greater sense of threat than gain-framed messages (Cox and Cox, 2001; Shen and Dillard, 2007). As is also explained in Chapter 8 on using frightening messages, messages which are perceived as threatening may evoke defensive cognitive reactions. This, in turn, may cause readers to dismiss your message entirely. Chapter 8 provides a more elaborate explanation of the cognitive mechanisms involved. For now, it is important to realise that gain frames do not evoke these processes and thus are a 'safe option' if you do not know how risky your target audience perceives your targeted behaviour to be for them.

This cognitive 'defensive' mechanism may be especially important when recipients do not feel capable of averting the threat by performing the recommended action. As noted in Chapters 7 and 8 such confidence in one's ability to perform a behaviour is known as self-efficacy (Bandura, 1986). It is important to consider the levels of self efficacy of your target audience in relation to the target behaviour in deciding what frame to use to strengthen written health messages. This can be ascertained through elicitation research (see Chapter 7). When self-efficacy is high, the threatening quality of loss-framed messages may not evoke defensive reactions and thus, still be effective. So we need to consider the perceived riskiness of a recommended action and the reader's likely self-efficacy in relation to its performance when selecting a loss or gain frame. Remember however, when in doubt, use a gain frame.

9.4 High self-efficacy matters

In Chapter 8, Ruiter and Kok argue that fear arousal should only be considered if recipients strongly believe in their abilities to avert a threat by performing the recommended action (that is, they have high self-efficacy). If, instead, recipients have low self-efficacy, a greater sense of threat (as communicated by fear appeal) may result in less message acceptance due to cognitive defensive mechanisms. Thus, the perception of threat might be similar for recipients with high and low self-efficacy, but their reactions may differ. More specifically, a high perceived threat can lead to defensiveness for recipients with low perceived efficacy and to effective persuasion for recipients with high perceived efficacy because the latter feel more able to cope with the threat.

Loss-framed messages have been found to evoke a greater sense of threat than gain-framed messages (Cox et al., 2006; Shen and Dillard, 2007). So loss-framed messages might be more persuasive than gain-framed messages because of the greater threat they entail, but this is only likely to be true for readers with high perceived efficacy. If a reader has a low self-efficacy, the induced feelings of threat from a loss frame might result in defensive cognitive processing of the message such that it has no persuasive effect. Recent studies have confirmed that self-efficacy influences the effectiveness of gain- versus loss-framed health promotion messages. For example, in one study participants with high self-efficacy were more motivated to quit smoking after reading a loss-framed message about the costs of not quitting than after reading a gain-framed message about the benefits of quitting or no message at all. However, for participants with low self-efficacy, the loss-framed messages were not more effective than the gain-framed message (Van 't Riet et al., 2008). In further studies involving people with high self-efficacy towards performing regular self-examination to detect skin cancer and reducing salt consumption to prevent hypertension respectively, loss frames were again found to be more effective than gain frames. However, for people with low self-efficacy, again no advantage was found for the loss frame (Van 't Riet et al., 2010a, 2010b).

Surprisingly, in our last study testing the effects of message framing under high levels of self-efficacy, we found a gain frame to be more effective than a loss frame in motivating people to replace regular meat with ecologically produced meat. Again, no advantage was found for either frame in people with low self-efficacy towards buying ecological meat (Werrij et al., 2001).

From the research described above, three conclusions can be drawn:

1   Message framing is only helpful in strengthening the persuasive effects of health messages if readers feel confident to perform the advocated health behaviour. If people lack this confidence (and so report low self-efficacy beliefs), message framing does not seem to make a difference to the persuasive impact of health messages. For low self-efficacy readers, gain-framed messages are recommended because they are less likely to result in defensive rejection of the message.
2   Loss-frames may be more effective if the target group have high self-efficacy and also regard the recommended action as risky. However, exceptions to this rule might be found, as you have seen above.
3   If good elicitation research has been conducted you may know your readers' likely response to loss- or gain-framed messages. If not, then a small pilot study in the pre-testing stage of the health message will be useful to gather evidence of how readers respond to loss versus gain frames.

9.5 Establishing a 'fit' between receiver, message and frame

Some authors (Cesario et al., 2004; Lee and Aaker, 2004) propose that increased persuasion will occur when readers perceive a 'fit' between the focus of the message and its frame (i.e., gain- or loss-frame). Health messages can adopt a 'promotion' or 'prevention' focus, by stressing the gains that will be attained or the losses that will be prevented by performing the recommended action. For example, consider an advertisement about grape juice. A promotion-focused message would concentrate on the energy-providing properties of the juice e.g.: 'Preliminary medical research suggests that drinking purple grape juice may contribute to a greater energy!' A prevention-focused message on the other hand, stressing the disease-preventing properties of the juice could look like: 'Preliminary medical research suggests that drinking purple grape juice may contribute to healthy cardiovascular function.'

Gain-framed messages are expected to be more effective when the message highlights promotion concerns. Loss-framed messages on the other hand, are expected to be more effective when the message highlights prevention concerns. Indeed, research revealed that if the message is promotion-focused, gain-framed messages ('get energised') are more persuasive than loss-framed messages ('don't miss out on getting energised'). In contrast, when the message is prevention-focused, loss-framed messages ('don't miss out on preventing clogged arteries') are more persuasive than gain-framed messages ('prevent clogged arteries') (Lee and Aaker, 2004). *Thus, increased persuasion seems to occur when message receivers perceive a 'fit' between the focus of the message on either gains that can be attained or losses that can be prevented (i.e., promotion or prevention) and its frame (i.e., gain or loss frame).*

9.6 How to frame messages: conclusions and recommendations

As this chapter illustrates, research on the effects of message framing is on-going and the underlying mechanisms are complex. We have discussed the perceptions of the behaviour as safe versus risky, self-efficacy, and the function of the promoted behaviour, as three particularly noteworthy contexts that may change – or moderate – (see Chapter 7) – the persuasive effects of message framing. Other factors have also been explored as potential moderators of message framing, among which the readers' level of information processing, their approach- or avoidance orientation (BIS/BAS), perceived behavioural norms, attitudinal ambivalence, ease of imagination, mood, level of education, intention to engage in the recommended behaviour, and source credibility. However, for some of these factors the evidence was limited to a single study or to a single health behaviour. For others, implications for message design were very complex. It seems that, as yet, not enough studies are available to draw conclusions relevant to those writing health promoting texts. These factors are therefore not included in this chapter as our primary aim was to provide evidence based practical guidelines for health professionals. However, the three contexts discussed above deserve your attention when thinking about the use of message framing to strengthen your health promotion materials – see Table 9.2.

In particular, use loss-framed messages which emphasise what is to be lost by not undertaking the recommended health behaviour if *all* of the following apply:

1   Readers *do* expect the recommended behaviour to involve *risk*.
2   Readers' self-efficacy regarding the recommended behaviour is *high*.
3   It makes more sense to emphasise the prevention of losses (prevention focus) rather than the attainment of gains.

Table 9.2 When to use gain- or loss-framed messages

Factor affecting framing effectiveness	Use gain-framed messages	Use loss-framed messages
Perceived riskiness	When readers perceive the recommended behaviour to be low in risk	When readers perceive the recommended behaviour to be high in risk
Self-efficacy	When readers' self-efficacy beliefs are unknown or low	Only when readers have high self-efficacy beliefs (but pilot test)
Message fit	When the message focuses on attaining gains	When the message focuses on preventing losses

Use gain-framed messages which emphasise what is to be gained by undertaking the recommended health behaviour if *any* of the following apply:

1 Readers *do not* expect the recommended behaviour to involve risk; or
2 Recipients' self-efficacy regarding the recommended behaviour is unknown or low, or
3 The message emphasises the attainment of gains (promotion focus) rather than the prevention of losses; or
4 You want to avoid any risk of eliciting defensive reactions in your readers.

References

Abhyankar, P., O'Connor, D.B. and Lawton, R. (2008) 'The role of message framing in promoting MMR vaccination: evidence of a loss frame advantage', *Psychology, Health & Medicine*, 13: 1–16.

Apanovitch, A.M., McCarthy, D. and Salovey, P. (2003) 'Using message framing to motivate HIV testing among low-income, ethnic minority women', *Health Psychology*, 22: 60–7.

Bandura, A. (1986) *Social Foundations of Thought and Action*. Englewood Cliffs, NJ: Prentice-Hall.

Cesario, J., Grant, H. and Higgins, E.T. (2004) 'Regulatory fit and persuasion: transfer from "Feeling Right"', *Journal of Pers Soc Psychol*, 86: 388–404.

Cox, A.D., Cox, D. and Zimet, G. (2006) 'Understanding consumer responses to product risk information', *Journal of Marketing*, 70, 79–91.

Cox, D. and Cox, A.D. (2001) 'Communicating the consequences of early detection: the role of evidence and framing', *Journal of Marketing*, 65: 91–103.

Detweiler, J.B., Bedell, B.T., Salovey, P., Pronin, E. and Rothman, A.J. (1999) 'Message framing and sunscreen use: gain-framed messages motivate beachgoers', *Health Psychology*, 18: 189–196.

Writing health communication

Lee, A.Y. and Aaker, J.L. (2004) 'Bringing the frame into focus: the influence of regulatory fit on processing fluency and persuasion', *Journal of Personality and Social Psychology*, 86: 205–18.

O'Keefe, D.J. and Jensen, J.D. (2007) 'The relative effectiveness of gain-framed loss framed messages for encouraging disease prevention behaviors: a meta-analytic review', *Journal of Health Communication*, 12: 623–44.

O'Keefe, D.J. and Jensen, J.D. (2009) 'The relative persuasiveness of gain-framed and loss-framed messages for encouraging disease detection behaviors: a meta-analytic review', *Journal of Communication*, 59, 296–316.

Rothman, A.J. and Salovey, P. (1997) 'Shaping perceptions to motivate healthy behaviour: the role of message framing', *Psychological Bulletin*, 121: 3–19.

Shen, L. and Dillard, J.P. (2007) 'The influence of behavioral inhibition/approach systems and message framing on the processing of persuasive health messages', *Communication Research*, 34, 433–67.

Tversky, A. and Kahneman, D. (1981) 'The framing of decisions and the psychology of choice', *Science*, 211: 453–8.

van 't Riet, J., Ruiter, R.A.C., Werrij, M.Q. and De Vries, H. (2008) 'The influence of self-efficacy on the effects of framed health messages', *European Journal of Social Psychology*, 38: 800–9.

van 't Riet, J., Ruiter, R.A.C., Smerecnik, C. and De Vries, H. (2010a) 'Examining the influence of self-efficacy on message-framing effects: reducing salt consumption in the general population', *Basic and Applied Social Psychology*, 32: 165–72.

van 't Riet, J., Ruiter, R.A.C., Werrij, M. and De Vries, H. (2010b) 'Self-efficacy moderates message-framing effects: the case of skin-cancer detection', *Psychology and Health*, 25: 339–49.

Werrij, M.Q., Ruiter, R.A.C., Van 't Riet, J. and De Vries, H. (2011) 'Self-efficacy as a potential moderator of the effects of framed health messages', *Journal of Health Psychology*, 16: 199–207.

10

Computer-tailoring of health promotion messages

Johannes Brug and Anke Oenema

Tailoring has been defined as 'any combination of information or change strategies intended to reach one specific person, based on characteristics that are unique to that person, related to the outcome of interest …[and] derived from an individual assessment' (Kreuter et al., 1999).

In other words, the message is tailored to match the needs of a particular reader on the basis of a prior assessment of that person. Research suggests that when health promotion messages are tailored to match personal characteristics, they are perceived to be more interesting and personally relevant and, importantly, are more likely to be effective in changing cognitions and behaviour. Tailored messages can be delivered face-to-face and using computer-based expert systems. Computer-tailored interventions mimic tailoring in face-to-face counselling, providing information and advice based on an individual's needs and characteristics, including their current levels of knowledge, their motivation and their behaviour skills. This ensures personal relevance. The World-Wide Web and mobile Internet systems present excellent opportunities to provide people with tailored health education messages when and where they are most needed.

In this chapter, we will describe the rationale for using computer-tailoring and provide an outline of what is necessary to deliver computer-tailored health promotion. We will describe how computer-tailored interventions are developed and implemented. We will explain how such interventions have been evaluated and assess how effective they have been. Finally, we will discuss how the World-Wide Web can support delivery of computer-tailored health education and consider future developments in computer-tailoring. We will use computer-tailored nutrition education interventions to illustrate these points.

Learning Outcomes

After reading this chapter, you should be able to:

1 Understand and use a model of planned health promotion including Intervention Mapping.
2 Judge when tailored health education is needed and appropriate.

3 Judge when, and for whom, computer-tailoring is likely to be most effective.
4 Understand and follow a series of steps involved in constructing computer-
  tailored health promotion interventions.
5 Discuss the effectiveness of computer-tailoring in health education.

10.1 Advantages of personally-tailored messages

We are likely to enhance our health and longevity if we do not smoke, only drink alcohol in moderate amounts; exercise for at least 30 minutes per day; eat a diet low in calories, saturated fat, and salt, but high in fibre, fruits and vegetables; have only protected sex; participate in cancer screening pro- grammes, and get vaccinated for a range of infectious diseases. These are just some of the behaviour patterns recommended by official health authorities. Many campaigns have been launched to promote such behaviour patterns. At the same time, contradictory messages are broadcast in advertisements and product placements used to sell various products. It is not easy for the general public to know which messages are relevant and which ones can be ignored. For example, judging whether a nutrition message advising reduction of satu- rated fat is important for *you*, requires you to understand what saturated fat is and to know if your present diet provides too much saturated fat. If your diet is already low in fat, there is no need to change but most people do not know how much saturated fat they eat. Therefore, most people do not know if, or how well, they comply with health behaviour recommendations. Moreover, they do not know which behaviour changes are necessary or appropriate for them so that they achieve recommended targets. Providing information and advice that is personally relevant to the recipient enables him/her to know immediately how relevant a health message is to them and what they need to do to meet recommendations.

Computer-tailored interventions embed diagnostic and educational exper- tise in a computerised expert system. They can provide a person with informa- tion, advice, feedback and persuasive messages that are based on that individual's characteristics. Relevant characteristics, including physiological or biomedical risk factors, attitudes, normative beliefs, their perceived barriers to change, their self-efficacy, their intention to change and their current behav- ioural patterns can all be assessed and used to tailor messages. An important advantage of computer tailoring for health promoters is that personally-relevant information increases attention to the message (see Chapter 4) so that mes- sages are processed more intensively (Ruiter et al., 2006). This means the message is more likely to be remembered and so is more likely to influence future actions.

Computer tailoring has been used by health educators and health promotion agencies and so became a focus of evaluative research (De Vries and Brug, 1999).

Computer-tailoring of health promotion messages

Research suggests that computer-tailored interventions are more effective than their non-tailored equivalents (Kroeze et al., 2006; Noar et al., 2007).

10.2 An outline model of planned health promotion

Figure 10.1 presents an outline model of planned promotion of population health (Brug et al., 2005). According to this model, the first step in health promotion planning is the identification of a health problem that is serious and prevalent enough to justify spending time, money and other resources on developing and implementing an intervention. In the second step, the specific behavioural and environmental risk factors contributing to the health problem should be identified, as well as population groups who are exposed to these risk factors (see also a description of Intervention Mapping in Chapter 7). The third step in planned health promotion is to investigate the individual and environmental determinants or antecedents of exposure to risk factors. This planning phase should identify as precisely as possible why particular people in the population engage in risk behaviour and what could instigate behaviour change towards more healthy habits (see also Chapter 4). If applied to nutrition behaviour, this determinant analysis should, for example, establish why people eat too much saturated fat and whether such determinants differ in relation to gender, age and education.

In the fourth step, interventions should be developed that target the most important and most easily-modifiable behavioural determinants, being as specific as possible in matching content to antecedents of the target behaviour (see Chapters 4 and 5). Finally, in the fifth and final step, interventions should be implemented and disseminated in such a way that the people who most need intervention (among the target population) are reached in a manner which optimises intervention effectiveness.

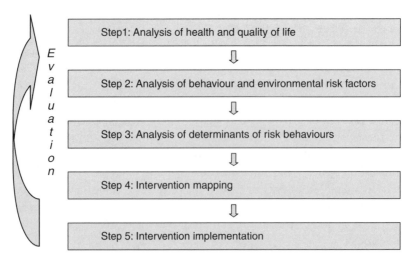

Figure 10.1   An overview model of planned health promotion

Writing health communication

10.3 Generic, targeted and tailored health promotion

10.3.1 Limits of generic health promotion

Most health education is generic. Using a one-size-fits-all approach, a particular educational intervention is developed for a large population group. Applying the model in Figure 10.1 to such generic health education, we should first establish which health problems are important for that group, which risk behaviours represent the most serious health risks in this population and which determinants of these risk behaviours are on average the most important. Such determinants could include cognitions such as attitudes, norms and self-efficacy (see Chapter 4). However the problem we face is that there may be a wide variety of relevant behaviour patterns and a similarly large range of determinants of those behaviours among the population. Computer-tailoring may be especially helpful when promoting complex behaviours such as nutrition and physical activity where wide variations exist in people's awareness, attitudes, intentions to change and behaviour patterns.

Consider an example: heart disease is a major burden of disease in most Western countries, including the Netherlands. Intake of too much saturated fat has been defined as a risk factor for heart disease, and food consumption research in the Netherlands has shown that saturated fat intake was too high for many Dutch adults. These facts led to the development of a nationwide health education campaign to reduce saturated fat intake among Dutch adults in the 1990s. Nutrition behaviour determinant studies show that taste preferences are of great importance for food choice, and additional research indicated that many people in the Netherlands thought that low fat foods and meals do not taste good. The 'Let op Vet' ('Fat Watch') campaign was developed and launched. In the early years, the campaign aimed to reduce fat consumption by trying to convince Dutch adults that low fat foods and meals can taste as good as higher fat ones. This was a sensible approach because, for a majority of the population, heart disease was an important health risk and, for a majority of this at-risk group, a high saturated fat diet was an important risk factor. Moreover, doubts about the tastiness of low fat food had been identified as a widespread barrier to behavioural change.

Nonetheless, this campaign may not have appealed to a large number of at-risk individuals for a variety of reasons. Some recipients might not eat too much saturated fat – or may not believe that they eat too much. Even if these people are persuaded that high saturated fat intake is a risk factor, they are unlikely to see it as relevant to them. Smoking and lack of physical activity are two other risk behaviours of importance. If a person does not eat much fat, but does not get enough physical activity, they may be more interested in messages about physical activity. In addition, some recipients may already be convinced that low fat food can taste good, or may feel that taste is less important than health considerations. For these people motivation, ability and opportunity to change (rather than beliefs about taste) may be more important to change

Computer-tailoring of health promotion messages

(Brug et al., 2005). Lack of motivation to reduce one's fat intake may, for some, be based on beliefs about the taste of low fat food, but motivation may also be low because of higher perceived costs or lower convenience of low fat eating, or, additionally, because of the perceived lack of social approval in lowering fat intake. Another group of recipients may have been motivated to change, but lacked the skills (e.g., cooking skills) or confidence to translate their motivation into dietary changes. Finally, some recipients may not have the economic or social resources in their environments to provide opportunities to change.

Often, a range of behaviour patterns may contribute to a given health problem in a certain population and, for each of these behaviours, a series of individual determinants (including cognitions such as attitudes and normative beliefs) may be relevant. Generic interventions cannot easily address such a range of different change targets and may risk presenting information and messages which are not relevant to many of the target group. If, however, the determinants of a specific dietary behaviour pattern differ very little between people in a certain population, then there is no need to use individual tailoring. In such a population, well-designed generic materials that address general determinants will be personally relevant for most of the target audience. Kreuter, Oswald, Bull and Clark (2000b) found evidence that when generic materials fitted well with the determinants and information needs of the majority of recipients the impact of generic materials was as good or better as that of tailored information. Thus, in populations in which health behaviour patterns differ little, there is no need to tailor messages.

10.3.2 Targeted health promotion: a step forward

As we noted in Chapters 4 and 5, various attempts have been made to match the content of health promotion messages more closely to behavioural determinants in target populations. Most of these attempts are based on *target-group segmentation*. This involves identifying at-risk sub-populations who are more homogeneous in their relevant risk behaviours and behavioural determinants. Conducting elicitation research (see Chapter 6) and carefully targeting the content of health promotion messages to such sub-groups can enhance the efficiency and effectiveness of health promotion over and above what can be achieved using generic messages. Group segmentation is often based on socio-demographic characteristics, such as age, gender or level of education. Even this approach cannot, however, match messages to the needs of individual recipients.

10.3.3 Individually-tailored health promotion

Individually-tailored health education is the ultimate goal of target-group segmentation; it matches the message to the individual recipients' personal characteristics. If a population does not exhibit much variety in risk behaviour patterns or important behavioural determinants, tailoring is not necessary. However, for most important health risks, a range of health risk behaviours are implicated, and a wide variety of individually-relevant behavioural determinants operate to

Writing health communication

sustain these risky behaviour patterns. Personal counselling is too time-consuming and too expensive to apply to population-level change. Computer-tailoring provides a way to target health promotion messages precisely at individualised change across large numbers of people at relatively low costs.

In computer-tailoring, evidence-based, and theory-informed medical, behavioural and health educational expertise is embedded in computer software. Existing expertise is translated into a set of algorithms that defines who gets what message at what time. Once such a system has been developed, it can be implemented and distributed widely so that expert, tailored health promotion can be provided in settings and at times when no expert health educator is available. This not only means that tailored health education becomes available for much larger groups than is possible using face-to-face counselling, it also means that expert, tailored health education can be made available at the most appropriate times and places.

Consider two examples. Medical doctors are often regarded as the most trustworthy and expert source of health information, including health behaviour change advice. However, doctors are often not experts on health behaviour, may not be well trained in health education skills and are required to conduct consultations that may be too short to allow time for individually-tailored health education. Computer-tailored health education systems in waiting rooms of doctors' surgeries, or available through their websites, which are actively supported and endorsed by doctors can combine the authority of the medical professional with the health education expertise embedded in the computer software. Studies have shown that computer-tailored health education offered through family doctors can be effective (Brug et al., 1999). However, when introducing computer-tailoring into organisational settings, it is important to anticipate knock-on effects such as the need for new staff training or changes in how work is organised. These may create initial resistance and subsequent organisational change processes will need to be managed if such systems are to be integrated effectively (Sciamanna et al., 2004).

A second type of application is at so-called 'point-of-choice' settings. For example, choices about food and nutrition are often made in restaurants and supermarkets. Computer-tailoring, especially when applied with mobile, Internet technology, allows the provision of tailored feedback anywhere and at any time, including such point-of-choice settings. For example, it is not difficult to foresee mobile phone 'apps' which could deliver personalised advice and persuasion at meal times, when shopping or other critical choice points.

10.4 How is computer-tailoring achieved?

Developing a computer-tailored intervention begins with making an intervention plan which sets out the specific goals of the intervention (Kreuter et al., 2000a). This will specify: (1) the target group; (2) the behaviour change targets; (3) important behavioural determinants that need to be targeted; and (4) how these determinants will be addressed by computer-tailored messages. It is critical that computer-tailored interventions are carefully planned and developed and

Computer-tailoring of health promotion messages

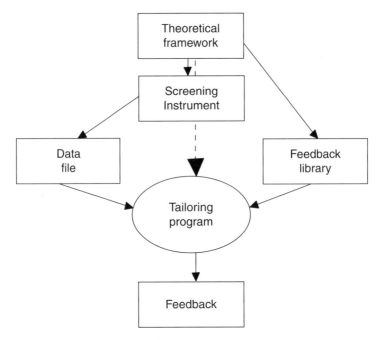

Figure 10.2   Key components of computer-tailored health promotion

based on the best available research and applicable theoretical insights. There is extensive evidence that careful theory-inspired and evidence-based planning increases the likelihood that the intervention will be effective (see Chapter 6).

The components of the computer program can be captured in six core elements (see Figure 10.2 above). These include:

- a theoretical framework;
- a screening or diagnostic instrument;
- a database system that stores the individual responses to the screening instrument;
- a message library containing feedback messages which match all relevant screening result variations;
- a computer program that defines 'tailoring algorithms' to select the appropriate message from the feedback library for any given response to the screening instrument;
- a format to coherently present and deliver the selected feedback messages to the respondent.

These core elements will be described in more detail below.

10.4.1 The theoretical framework

The theoretical framework is the foundation of the computer-tailored program. Using a theoretical framework ensures that the intervention targets the most important determinants of the behaviours identified by previous research.

Potentially important behavioural determinants are described in a range of health behaviour theories (see Chapter 7). Determinants may include awareness of risk behaviours, attitudes, normative beliefs, self-efficacy and intentions. The theoretical framework determines: (1) which questions need to be asked in the screening instrument; (2) which individual characteristics will be used to tailor messages; (3) the type, content and tone of the set of feedback messages which need to be available to the computer; and (4) how the tailoring algorithms should be defined. Most computer-tailored interventions have adopted theoretical frameworks that focus especially on individual-level motivation and ability-related health behaviour determinants, and so define change targets of this type (e.g., that promote positive attitudes or bolster self-efficacy). However, in recent years some interventions have been developed that include environmental opportunities as tailoring variables. So a key starting point is to develop a theoretical framework that best explains the targeted behaviour. This ensures that the relevant determinants will be targeted by the intervention. A theoretical framework can be based on insights and elements from established theories.

10.4.2 The screening instrument

The screening or diagnostic instrument assesses information on an individual's status on important biomedical factors (e.g., body mass index, cholesterol levels, blood pressure) as well as behaviour(s) and behavioural determinants defined in the theoretical framework. The information from the screening instrument is input that generates individualised computer-tailored feedback and advice. Using data provided by respondents during screening, the tailoring program selects only those feedback messages that match the characteristics of each individual respondent. In addition to information on behaviours and determinants, the screening instrument is also used to assess background characteristics, such as name, address, age, gender, educational level, or cultural norms, when such factors are important for further tailoring and personalising the message (Brug, 1999; Dijkstra and De Vries, 1999; Kreuter et al., 2000a). In most cases, developing a screening or diagnostic instrument means developing a questionnaire that assesses information about all characteristics which may be used to tailor messages. The screening instrument should be designed in such a way that it assesses these characteristics in a valid and reliable way and in sufficient detail, since the quality and the specificity of the tailored feedback depend on the specificity, validity and reliability of the personal assessment. This may mean using previously validated measures and employing a questionnaire-design expert. In most computer-tailored interventions to date, screening instruments consist of print or electronic, self-administered questionnaires (Noar et al., 2007). However, more objective information such as cholesterol level as an indicator of saturated fat intake, accelerometer data for physical activity, measured height, weight and waist circumference for weight management behaviours, or information from medical records can also be used as diagnostic information.

Consider the 'FATain'tPHAT' intervention, a computer-tailored program for adolescents that aimed at prevention of excessive weight gain (Ezendam et al., 2007). This program promoted behaviour change to avoid unnecessary weight gain, such as reducing snack foods, soft drinks and sedentary behaviours, as well as increasing fruit, vegetable and fibre intake, and physical activity. The precaution adoption process model (PAPM; Weinstein, 1988) and the theory of planned behaviour (TPB; Ajzen, 1991, see Chapter 6) were used as the theoretical frameworks to identify important determinants of these behaviours. The PAPM suggests that awareness of one's personal risk behaviour is a crucial prerequisite of motivation to change and that personal and normative behavioural feedback are behaviour change techniques that can promote such motivation.

Based on these theoretical frameworks, we included an assessment of all the specific target behaviours, as well as awareness of each risk behaviour, attitudes, subjective norm beliefs, perceived behavioural control and intention towards changing each relevant behaviour. We needed to be able to personalise information by using a person's name in the feedback messages and to match the information to the gender of the adolescents. So, first name and gender were included in the screening questionnaire. The program was web-based and all specific behaviours were addressed in separate modules that could be completed separately. Overall then, separate web-based questionnaires were developed for each relevant behaviour, and feedback messages were provided after the completion of each questionnaire.

10.4.3 The database system

A database system to store messages matching individual responses to the screening instrument is also required. Data from electronic assessment methods, such as web-based questionnaires, can be directly imported to such databases, but printed questionnaires need to be scanned or manually entered into an electronic format first. The data must be stored so that it can be directly matched to the characteristics used by the tailoring algorithms. Sometimes this requires calculation of new, composite measures from a number of questions in the screening questionnaire, such as, for example, calculation of a saturated fat intake measure based on a series of food frequency questions. The data in the database should preferably also be suitable for data analysis, i.e. in a format that can be used by software packages for statistical analyses so that the data can also be used for intervention evaluation. Health promoting agencies will need a programmer to help unless they adopt existing computer-tailoring software that can be customised to develop an entire computer-tailored program (including a database).

10.4.4 The message library

The message library contains feedback messages that match all possible responses to the tailoring characteristics assessed in the screening instrument. These feedback messages contain the educational elements that are needed to change the important behavioural determinants, taking account of individual characteristics. In the FATain'tPHAT, program, for example, using a theoretical framework based on the PAPM and the TPB, personal feedback and persuasive messages about determinants of dietary and physical activity were included; for example, feedback about how one's own soft drink intake compares to dietary recommendations and intake of peers. All adolescents would receive a message that provided feedback about how many soft drinks they consumed and how this compared to the 'norm' of a maximum of two glasses of soft drinks each day. The content and the tone of these messages differed according to how much the adolescent drank. Other sets of messages included, for example, factual information about certain aspects of the risk behaviour and its consequences. These were delivered to adolescents who were identified as lacking such knowledge by the screening process. For those who did not see the advantages of reducing soft drink intake, messages promoting a positive attitude towards reducing soft drink intake were included. As we have seen in Chapter 4, it is important that the content of such messages corresponds precisely to the change target specified by the theoretical framework (see Box 6.2).

As we have noted in Chapters 3 and 4 such messages need to be easy to understand and easy to use. Messages also need to be precisely targeted to the change targets specified by the theoretical framework and need to attract the attention of the target group (see Chapter 4). Messages do not necessarily include only textual information. They can also contain graphics, drawings, pictures, and, for interventions delivered in interactive formats, spoken text, music, video, web-links or animations.

It is important not to underestimate the time it takes to develop message libraries. In projects we have been involved in, more than 1000 feedback messages were written, accompanied by an even higher number of tailoring algorithms. Sufficient time must be budgeted for when planning such development work.

10.4.5 The tailoring program

The next step in the development of a computer-tailored program is writing tailoring algorithms that link individuals' responses to the screening instrument to the appropriate feedback/educational messages. In the simplest case, these algorithms state that 'if a participant gave answer x to question y, then message z has to be selected'. Algorithms become more complex when a feedback message is selected based on answers to different questions in the screening instrument or on combinations of tailoring characteristics – which is often desirable.

The tailoring algorithms are the heart of the tailoring program. Informed by the theoretical framework, they define what feedback messages have to be provided to people with particular characteristics, at what time. When all algorithms have been defined, a professional programmer has to develop the computer program that automates the process of selecting the appropriate messages. Alternatively, some

Computer-tailoring of health promotion messages

computer tailoring software enables health promotion professionals (without programming expertise) to customise existing algorithms into a bespoke program.

10.4.6 Message delivery

The final and crucial element of the tailoring program is the delivery of selected messages to recipients. Messages can be delivered as printed documents such as letters, newsletters or magazines, as emails, in spoken text or in short text messages using mobile phones – or in interactive, web-based formats.

Printed computer tailoring typically uses written surveys and delivers written messages (based on the individual survey results) in the form of personal letters or newsletters sent by mail. This procedure requires days or weeks. It is also more expensive than generic nutrition education, since it requires at least some handling of the survey questionnaires and the feedback letters. On the other hand, it allows messages to be delivered to recipients from a trusted source. This may enhance its credibility and allows users to read it as many times as they wish and to share it with others.

Using interactive technology has lower costs, less time between screening and feedback, and greater interactivity. For example, recipients can email 'experts' or participate in on-line discussion forums and/or chat sessions. This format can use attention-grabbing and educational visuals and employ a wider range of behaviour change techniques than most letters of newsletters. Moreover, participants can enter data more flexibly; for example, when using mouse clicks, a keyboard or voice recording, feedback can be provided almost immediately on the (computer) screen. This format is also appreciated by some target audiences such as young people. An early study using a web-based computer-tailored system showed that respondents who received interactive computer-tailored feedback appreciated their information more, were more aware of their fat intake levels and were more motivated to reduce their fat intake than respondents who received non-tailored information (Oenema et al., 2005), although this did not compare web-based and printed tailoring.

Regardless of the message format, it is important that messages are presented in a coherent and easy to follow sequence in an appropriate and attractive layout (see Chapters 3–5). Electronic delivery formats (such as websites) allow for greater flexibility but the choice of format will depend on the preferences of the target audience and budget constraints.

10.4.7 Pre-testing

Once all the elements of the computer tailoring program have been developed and organised, the program needs to be extensively tested for accuracy, acceptability, ease of use and ease of understanding by the target population. *Extensive pre-testing of the computer-tailored program is of crucial importance.* The developers must ensure that the program generates accurate, helpful and relevant messages to the right people at the right time. In addition, for web-based programs or other interactive delivery formats, it is important to test whether the program works properly outside the setting where it was created. Members of the target group need to be involved in pre-testing the program, to check if they can easily use the program, appreciate it and find it personally relevant. After appropriate adaptations to the program, it is ready for implementation and evaluation.

10.5 Does computer-tailoring work?

Several reviews of the scientific literature have demonstrated that tailored printed materials are more effective than standard health education messages (Brug et al., 2005). A meta-analysis by Noar et al. (2007) considered 57 interventions targeting a broad range of health behaviours and found that interventions targeting cervix and breast cancer screening, smoking cessation, dietary change and physical activity were effective, across studies.

In a systematic review of 30 evaluations, Kroeze et al. (2006) found that most interventions provided tailored feedback on the current behaviour of recipients and many included persuasive messages targeting benefits of and barriers to change and self-efficacy. Most interventions used single contacts, that is, one tailored letter, brochure or interactive feedback opportunity, but some studies investigated the effects of interventions that provided multiple tailored feedback messages, ranging from two to fifteen sessions. Eleven of 14 fat-reduction intervention evaluations testing short-term effects, showed a significant positive effect in favour of tailored interventions, either in comparison to a non-tailored intervention or no intervention.

Only two studies investigated longer-term follow-up and neither showed significant positive effects. In six out of ten studies on fruit and vegetable consumption and three out of four evaluations of interventions targeting fibre consumption, positive effects were reported. Two out of five evaluations of interventions designed to promote physical activity reported significant differences in favour of the tailored intervention, while two other studies found negative effects. Thus, overall, there are mixed findings but some very positive outcomes.

10.5.1 For whom does computer tailoring work?

Because most computer-tailored nutrition interventions to date have used (rather extensive) questionnaires as the screening instrument and have provided respondents with written feedback, it has been argued that computer-tailored nutrition education may only work for highly educated or motivated recipients (Brug and Van Assema, 2000). Indeed, health communication in general has been found to be more effective among more educated groups. Moreover, unmotivated people may not be willing to complete the screening survey or may not (attentively) read and process the tailored messages since they experience no 'need to change' and therefore no reason to participate in the intervention.

Computer-tailoring of health promotion messages

Most studies evaluating the efficacy of computer-tailored nutrition education have been conducted among self-selected samples and this typically results in over-representation of female, motivated and more highly educated respondents, indicating that, like health communications in general, computer-tailored nutrition education appeals more to highly educated, motivated women. However, one of our own early tailoring studies was conducted in a workplace setting among a largely male employee population, and resulted in a 74 per cent participation rate and significant reductions in fat intake in the tailored group (Brug et al., 1996), indicating that men can be interested in personalised feedback and persuasion relevant to their diet. Further, in a few larger studies which have included sufficient numbers of men and less highly educated or non-motivated respondents, no gender-by-intervention interactions have been reported, meaning that computer-tailored interventions can be equally effective for men and women and those more or less well educated. One study reported on the impact of computer-tailored nutrition education among people not yet motivated to change and people with a relatively low educational level (Brug and Van Assema, 2000). Computer tailoring proved to be more effective among those not yet motivated to change than generic nutrition information. Furthermore, unmotivated recipients made up 34 per cent of participants, indicating that many people with low initial motivation to change do attend to personalised dietary feedback when it is provided. These results suggest that, at least for dietary fat reduction, unmotivated people may lack awareness rather than being uninterested in or resistant to making changes.

The positive effects of computer tailoring have been repeatedly found for less well educated recipients – who may need intervention most. For example, the Health Works for Women and FoodSmart studies were conducted successfully among lower income and minority women (Campbell et al., 1999). However, such studies have not included people with hardly any education. For very poorly educated groups, literacy issues may prohibit the use of any text-based intervention. However, for those with some reading ability, tailoring may be especially useful because there is less information to read and sift through, since information that is not personally relevant is eliminated.

10.6 Why are computer-tailored interventions more effective?

The mechanisms through which computer tailoring may work are not fully understood. However, various working mechanisms have been suggested, and at least partly supported by empirical evidence. Computer-tailored interventions are thought to attract more *attention* to the message and induce more *cognitive processing* of the information (see also Chapter 9). Individualised *feedback* provided through computer tailoring can enhance these processes.

10.6.1 Enhancing attention and cognitive processing

An intervention can only be effective when people pay sufficient attention to its contents. Various attributes of computer-tailored interventions are likely to result in improved attention to the message. First of all, personalisation of information improves attention. Personalisation can in part be achieved by including reference to personal characteristics in the feedback messages, such as, for example, mentioning the recipient's name or his/her age, sex, family members' names or other characteristics that are important to a recipient. Improved attention is also realised because tailored information only includes information that is relevant for a recipient, thus restricting the amount of information. Consequently, more attention can be paid to the information provided. Measuring brain activity data using an electroencephalogram (EEG), Ruiter et al. (2006) showed that computer-tailored nutrition education attracts more attention than generic, non-tailored nutrition education

Attention to a message is a prerequisite for cognitive change, but certainly not sufficient. Cognitive processing of the information is a further condition for achieving effects. The elaboration likelihood model (Petty and Cacioppo, 1986) postulates that there are two routes of information processing: a central route and a peripheral route. Central route information processing leads to stronger and more sustained changes in attitudes, and is therefore to be preferred. Such central route information processing is characterised by careful and thoughtful consideration of the information presented and is more likely to occur when people are motivated and able to process the information thoroughly. Motivation for central route processing is more likely when the information is perceived as personally relevant. Various studies indicate that computer-tailored information is centrally processed. These include process evaluation studies which have demonstrated that computer-tailored information is more likely to be fully read, discussed with others, and saved, compared to generic information (Brug et al., 1996; Kreuter et al., 2000a). In addition, it has been found that people who were exposed to computer-tailored weight loss materials generated more positive thoughts, more positive self-connection thoughts, more positive behavioural intention thoughts, and more positive self-assessment thoughts related to weight management and weight-loss behaviours, than participants exposed to generic information. Finally, the interactive nature of tailored messages may enhance cognitive processing; interactivity may lead to more involvement with the message and more active information processing.

10.6.2 The effects of feedback

The personalised feedback that can be provided in computer-tailored interventions is an important behaviour change technique. Feedback directly linked to personal knowledge of one's own behaviour and intentions is more personally salient and, therefore, more likely to elicit central route processing. Employment

Computer-tailoring of health promotion messages

of other behaviour change techniques such as the provision of normative feed-back may also be important to the success of computer tailoring (Oenema et al., 2005). Other behaviour change techniques frequently used include use of role models closely matched to characteristics of the recipient, personal goal setting, making personal action plans and provision of personalised feedback on progress towards achieving set goals (see Chapter 9).

10.7 The future of computer-tailored interventions

Two future developments in computer tailoring will be briefly discussed. First, the use of new technologies and, second, tailoring using new personal characteristics.

10.7.1 Use of new technologies

Web-delivered computer-tailored interventions can be combined with a variety of other technologies, such as e-mail, short text messaging (SMS) and Twitter and Internet social networking platforms. This can allow delivery of behaviour change techniques at times and places when they are most needed. For example, a recipient can be sent various different tailored text messages at pre-set risk times agreed in advance with the recipient. Furthermore, diagnostic data from new behaviour monitoring systems, such as accelerometers for assessing physical activity or shopping cards that register purchases can be inputted directly by the recipients to generate computer-tailored feedback that changes as the recipient makes progress towards their behaviour change goals. Web-based interventions can also direct recipients to selected web-based information resources or support groups (including peers striving to change the same behaviour patterns).

Use of the World-Wide Web also presents challenges for health promoters. The enormity of the Web, with its virtually unlimited amount of information, the limited possibilities to check the validity of the information, the sometimes doubtful sources of information, as well as the limitless opportunities to 'click' through to other websites on completely different topics, may all be barriers to accessing cred-ible and effective nutrition education messages. Consequently, the potential of Internet-based, interactive, tailored nutrition education has not been fully tested or exploited. The behaviour change effects of innovative applications must be carefully pre-tested before concluding that they will enhance intervention effectiveness.

10.7.2 Use of new tailoring characteristics

Computer tailoring may also be improved by measuring new individual differ-ences, and tailoring messages to these characteristics. Candidates include strength of habit, implicit attitudes, pre-existing self-regulation skills, self-determination processes, social networks and social support and perceptions of the physical and social environment.

Options for arranging peer support and direct interaction with peers are limited in computer-tailored interventions. Yet dietary habits are often not volitional or personally determined because food is often bought or prepared by others. Attempts have therefore been made to conduct family-based tailored nutrition education, in which different family members received tailored feedback and were encouraged to discuss their feedback, especially with the person responsible for cooking and shopping (De Bourdeaudhuij and Brug, 2000).

10.8 Conclusion

In this chapter we described what computer tailoring is, when it can be used effectively and how this can be achieved. Computer tailoring is complex to set up but once operational can be used to provide individualised health promotion at relatively low cost to large numbers of people. Personalised messages are more likely to be viewed as important and relevant. Personal messages are also more likely to be attended to and actively processed and so more likely to result in behaviour change. Reviews of the evaluative literature have shown that computer-tailored interventions are often more effective than generic health promotion interventions. Providing computer-tailored interventions is most likely to be effective when tackling complex behaviour patterns at population level, and when there is considerable variability between people both in terms of their behaviour and the determinants of that behaviour. It is critical to pre-test such systems, checking their accuracy, completeness, stability and effectiveness.

References

Ajzen, I. (1991) 'The theory of planned behavior', *Organizational Behavior and Human Decision Processes*, 50: 179–211.

Brug, J. (1999) 'Dutch research into the development and impact of computer-tailored nutrition education', *European Journal of Clinical Nutrition*, 53: S78–82.

Brug, J., Campbell, M. and Van Assema, P. (1999) 'The application and impact of computer-generated personalized nutrition education: a review of the literature', *Patient Education and Counseling*, 36: 145–56.

Brug, J., Oenema, A., and Ferreira, I. (2005) 'Theory, evidence and Intervention Mapping to improve behavior nutrition and physical activity interventions', *International Journal of Behavioral Nutrition and Physical Activity*, 2: 2.

Brug, J., Steenhuis, I.H.M., Van Assema, P., and De Vries, H. (1996) 'The impact of a computer-tailored nutrition intervention', *Preventive Medicine*, 25: 236–42.

Brug, J. and Van Assema, P. (2000) 'Differences in use and impact of computer-tailored fat-feedback according to stage of change and education', *Appetite*, 34: 285–93.

Campbell, M.K., Honess, L., Farrell, D., Carbone, E. and Brasure, M. (1999) 'Effects of a tailored multimedia nutrition education program for low income women receiving food assistance', *Health Education Research*, 14: 246–56.

De Bourdeaudhuij, I.D., and Brug, J. (2000) 'Tailoring dietary feedback to reduce fat intake: an intervention at the family level', *Health Education Research*, 15: 449–62.

De Vries, H. and Brug, J. (1999) 'Computer-tailored interventions to promote health promoting behaviours: an introduction to a new approach', *Patient Education and Counselling*, 36: 99–105.

Dijkstra, A. and De Vries, H. (1999) 'The development of computer-generated tailored interventions', *Patient Education and Counselling*, 36: 193–203.

Ezendam, N.P., Oenema, A., van de Looij-Jansen P.M. and Brug, J. (2007) 'Design and evaluation protocol of "FATaintPHAT", a computer-tailored intervention to prevent excessive weight gain in adolescents', *BMC Public Health*, 7: 324.

Kreuter, M.W., Bull, F.C., Clark, E.M. and Oswald, D.L. (1999) 'Understanding how people process health information: a comparison of tailored and untailored weight loss materials', *Health Psychology*, 18: 1–8.

Kreuter, M., Farrell, D., Olevitch. L. and Brennan L. (2000a) *Tailoring Health Messages: Customizing Communication with Computer Technology*. Mahwah, NJ: Lawrence Elbaum.

Kreuter, M.W., Oswald, D.L., Bull, F.C., and Clark, E.M. (2000b) 'Are tailored health education materials always more effective than non-tailored materials?' *Health Education Research*, 15: 101–11.

Kroeze, W., Werkman, A. and Brug, J. (2006) 'A systematic review of randomized trials on the effectiveness of computer-tailored education on physical activity and dietary behaviors', *Annals of Behavioral Medicine*, 31: 205–23.

Noar, S.M., Benac, C.M. and Harris, M.S. (2007) 'Does tailoring matter? Meta-analytic review of tailored print health behavior change interventions', *Psychological Bulletin*, 133: 673–93.

Oenema, A., Tan, F. and Brug, J. (2005) 'Short-term efficacy of a web-based computer-tailored nutrition intervention: main effects and mediators', *Annals of Behavioral Medicine*, 29: 54–63.

Petty, R.E. and Cacioppo, J.T. (1986) 'The elaboration likelihood model of persuasion', in L. Berkowitz (ed.), *Advances in Experimental Social Psychology*, vol. 19, New York: Academic Press, pp. 123–205.

Ruiter, R.A., Kessels, L.T., Jansma, B. and Brug J. (2006) 'Increased attention for computer-tailored health communications: an event-related potential study', *Health Psychology*, 25: 300–6.

Sciamanna, C.N., Marchs, B.H., Goldstein, M.G., Lawrence, K., Swartz, S., Block, B., Graham, A.L. and Ahern, D.K. (2004) 'Feasibility of incorporating computer tailored health behaviour communications in primary care settings', *Informatics in Primary Care*, 12: 40–8.

Weinstein, N.D. (1988) 'The precaution adoption process', *Health Psychology*, 7: 355–86.

Writing health communication

11

Conclusions and recommendations

Charles Abraham and Marieke Kools

11.1 A bite-sized summary

This final chapter provides a summary of the whole book. It does not matter if you are reading it immediately after Chapter 1 or after you have read many of the chapters. We highlight the key conclusions authors have reached and, in particular, the practical recommendations they have made for preparing written health promotion materials. We hope this brief summary allows you to assimilate the main points of the book in one bite-sized read. However, we have not been able to include all the practical recommendations here. The chapter is a sample of what the individual chapters offer – so please, when something interests you, return to the detailed contents pages to find detailed explanations and further recommendations.

11.2 Summary of Chapter 2 Designing easy-to-read text

In this chapter, James Hartley provides practical advice on how to lay out text so that it is easy to read. As he notes, if written materials are not read, then they cannot be persuasive or impact on health-related motivation or behaviour.

The chapter provides advice on how to select:

1 page size and orientation;
2 consistent spacing around a text to optimise understanding;
3 type-sizes and typefaces;
4 ways to emphasise and differentiate text (e.g., use of italics).

The chapter notes that page size and positioning are important and that, for example, a poster that is difficult to read from a distance may never be read.

Consistent and systematic spacing helps the reader to understand the structure of documents, helps them read faster and identify parts of the text that are most relevant to them. There is also some evidence that unjustified text may be easier to read for less able readers, including young children or older adults

The chapter points out that 12-point type with one-and-a-half line-spacing can be read by most people (including those with minor visual impairments) and compares various fonts.

Four key structural elements are recommended;

1   a detailed contents page;
2   a skeleton outlines for each chapter;
3   headings in the text;
4   a concluding summary.

The chapter concludes with a useful list of do's and don'ts. These include the following:

Do

• consider using unjustified text and *do* pre-test the text with a mixture of appropriate readers.

Do not
• over-use cues to emphasise text (especially capital letters, underlining and colour).

11.3 Summary of Chapter 3
Making written materials easy to understand

In this chapter, Marieke Kools makes the point that understanding the message is essential to facilitating behavioural change. The chapter focuses on enhancing the understanding of written text by taking account of cognitive mechanisms underpinning readers' comprehension. An important general rule is that only a limited number of concepts can be held active in working memory at any point in time. So it is important that:

1   not too many concepts are introduced in a particular section of text;
2   text and graphics should match up and are placed in close proximity to each other.

Research findings on several textual and graphical features are explained and good and bad examples of text and figure design are discussed. The chapter considers:

1   textual features that prepare readers for demanding text at a global/macro level or the local, micro level of the text;
2   graphic organisers that graphically integrate and summarise the main relationships between relatively abstract concepts outlined in the text;
3   icons that identify or emphasise different kinds of text;
4   illustrations that explain textual information visually, by showing important features and relationships. For example, the section on how to design illustrations, notes the following: procedural information that needs to be acted upon, should present a combination of illustrations in the form of simple line-drawings and

text. In general, comprehension of any complex information can be facilitated by use of line-drawings.

5 A careful analysis of materials may help determine which parts most need visual support and/or extended text.

6 Testing of instructions with novice users by observing their actions and subsequent re-design of text is recommended.

Finally, advice is provided on how to test the effectiveness of materials. For example, just asking readers if they understand may not be appropriate because readers may feel obliged to be positive to acknowledge the efforts of the text designers. The chapter explains how objective measures in which readers are asked to explain the meaning of the text can be employed.

11.4 Summary of Chapter 4
Making written materials easy to use

In this chapter, Marieke Kools explains the applied research field of 'cognitive ergonomics', which looks at the design of materials from a 'usability' perspective: how do people use your materials and how can you as a designer use this information to improve the 'usability' of your materials?

Capturing and focusing your readers' attention and helping them find specific information within your text is critical to the impact of the text. So too is understanding how readers perceive, understand and use your materials.

Usability is about understanding the structure of your materials. To help your reader understand your design, find information fast and feel positively about your materials, your materials should have high 'usability'. A series of usability factors are discussed, including ensuring that:

1 materials are flexible to the needs and wishes of various kinds of users;
2 materials are easy to learn;
3 materials require minimal working-memory and long-term memory loads;
4 materials provide a user guidance scheme.

Each piece of advice is described in detail and concrete do's and don't's are listed, for the design of print materials as well as websites. This chapter provides advice on testing the usability of your designs using objective measures. This may include using an experimental design with two groups of readers or an interview-based qualitative approach depending on time and financial constraints. A reassuring finding reported in the chapter is that with only four or five members of your target audience you may reveal up to 80 per cent of all potential usability problems within your materials. Several methods are described to test for the concrete usability characteristics of 'effectiveness', 'efficiency', 'learnability' and 'satisfaction'.

Conclusions and recommendations

11.5 Summary of Chapter 5
Using graphics effectively in text

In this chapter, Patricia Wright begins by discussing the communication purposes of text messages. She advises designers to consider carefully what each graphic communicates and how this augments the text itself. She notes that the purposes served by any particular graphic should be clear to the designer and that the graphic should be positioned carefully in the text to facilitate reading (see also Chapter 3). This chapter also reminds designers that graphics (like text) must be tailored to readers' knowledge (or lack of knowledge). For example, will your readers understand the symbols you use? In addition, the chapter emphasises that graphics do not replace clear writing and, if badly chosen, can undermine text messages. So, as is emphasised in Chapters 3 and 4, careful consideration, pre-testing and evaluation that explores readers' responses are important.

The chapter sets out a simple three-stage process for selecting graphics.

- Decide on the purpose of the graphic.
- Select a graphic style.
- Locate the graphics appropriately within the leaflet.

The chapter highlights communication purposes for graphics that are likely to enhance plain text. Graphics can encourage people to read text. They are useful when providing instructions (see also Chapter 3) and when explaining simultaneous or 'parallel' processes. They can also be very useful when explaining risk, probabilities and frequencies. Graphics can also arouse emotion but should be used cautiously in this role (see Chapter 8).

The chapter offers some key recommendations on how to select and use graphics. For example;

1   Consider line-drawings rather than photographs for clarity and for audience inclusiveness.
2   Keep the graphics simple, whether they are drawings, photographs or data charts.
3   Write captions that will help readers focus on the relevant part of the picture and interpret the graphic correctly.
4   Remember graphic representations must be culturally sensitive.

11.6 Summary of Chapter 6
Developing evidence-based content for health promotion materials

In this chapter, Charles Abraham argues that integrative theoretical frameworks and elicitation research can help match health promotion messages to the behavioural problems they address. Elicitation research involves investigation (for example, using interviews) into what the target audience already know, think and do. This chapter notes that health promotion texts are based on the assumption that:

1 We can identify (from research) which cognitions and preparatory actions are associated with the target behaviour.
2 Persuasive messages in health promotion texts directly target these cognitions and actions.
3 Readers are motivated to read and process these persuasive messages.

The chapter considers two integrative theoretical frameworks, the information motivation behavioural skills model and a framework which identifies core elements of motivation. The latter model emphasises a series of beliefs that may need to be changed in order to motivate readers to adopt a recommended health behaviour:

1 perceiving advantages of recommended behaviour change;
2 perceiving prevalence and acceptance of the behaviour among peers;
3 perceiving correspondence with self-image;
4 anticipating feeling good about adopting the behaviour;
5 believing that one can successfully perform the behaviour (self-efficacy).

The chapter shows how selection of antecedents of behaviour change from theoretical frameworks which draw upon a range of research can help specify what messages are needed in a particular health promotion text. This idea is developed in Chapter 7.

Finally, the chapter also notes that readers may be more or less motivated to read health promotion messages and considers ways in which motivation can be enhanced.

11.7 Summary of Chapter 7
Mapping change mechanisms onto behaviour change techniques: a systematic approach to promoting behaviour change through text

In this chapter, Charles Abraham recommends that designers answer the following questions before deciding on message content:

1 What is the problem that necessitates intervention?
2 Who needs to change?
3 What behaviours need to be change?
4 What change mechanisms need to be activated in order to promote changes in awareness, motivation and skills?

5   What behaviour change techniques can be used to activate these specific changes?
6   How can these behaviour change techniques be written into health promotion materials?

The author describes a planning process that links the nature of the behaviour change problem (which the written materials address) to the content of the messages included in the written materials. The chapter provides a list of 11 change processes which messages might target. Designers are encouraged to select change processes when answering question 4. For example, if our knowledge of the target group suggests that they lack self-efficacy, a key change process is likely to be – 'enhance self-efficacy'. In addition, the chapter also provides a menu of 40 behaviour change techniques grouped according to which of the 11 change processes they target. Designers are encouraged to consider selecting those that best suit to the needs of their target audience. Elicitation research, for example, observing or interviewing the target group may help in selection of change processes and behaviour change techniques.

Further, having identified 'enhance self-efficacy' as a key change process, designers might then select the behaviour change technique – 'use argument to boost self-efficacy'. They might then include messages such as: 'Just a little practice will allow you to handle and use condoms quickly.'

In addition, they might also select a behaviour change technique such as 'provide instruction'. In this case they might include a series of line-drawn graphics illustrating correct use, with captions explaining what each graphic means, such as, 'Place the condom on the tip of the erect penis with the rolled side out.'

This chapter also recommends that evaluation should feed into future design. Consequently, evaluation should discover how effective materials were, for whom and how they were delivered or used in practice.

11.8 Summary of Chapter 8
Planning to frighten people? Think again!

In this chapter Robert Ruiter and Gerjo Kok consider the use of frightening messages (or fear appeals) in health promotion. They acknowledge the popularity of fear appeals but also present evidence indicating that, unless carefully designed, fear appeals may be ineffective or even confirm recipients' rationalisations of risky health-related behaviour.

The chapter explains that a well-designed fear appeal should communicate two messages:

1 There is a serious threat (e.g., lung cancer) to which the recipient is susceptible (e.g., 'smoking cigarettes puts you at risk of lung cancer').

2 There is an effective way to avoid the undesirable consequence (e.g., quitting smoking) and this is something the recipient can easily do (e.g., 'free smoking cessation groups help the majority of attendees to quit').

The authors point out that many fear appeals focus on the first idea and either omit or fail to emphasise the second. This is worrying because without the second message recipients feel threatened but may have little confidence that they can protect themselves. Faced with a serious threat which they cannot protect against, recipients may defend themselves psychologically by denying the reality of the threat. They may question the credibility of the message or claim that they have special immunity (e.g., 'my father smoked all his life and never had lung cancer'). When this happens, they are either no more likely, or even less likely, to change their behaviour in line with the recommendation! '

The authors emphasise the importance of giving recipients confidence that they can avoid the threat by boosting self-efficacy in relation to the recommended behaviour. They offer advice on approaches other that fear appeals and correct use of fear appeals.

11.9 Summary of Chapter 9
Message framing

In this chapter, Marieke Werrij, Robert Ruiter, Jonathan van 't Riet and Hein de Vries describe the principle of message framing, which proposes that the precise wording of messages can have an impact on the persuasiveness of that message. Generally, two kinds of message frames can be developed, both include the same information but phrase the outcomes in terms of gains or losses.

1 *Gain frames* emphasise potential gains of the target behaviour, for example, 'if you maintain a healthy weight, you reduce the risk of getting cancer.'
2 *Loss frames* stress the losses that follow from on engaging in the target behaviour, for example, 'if you are overweight or obese, you increase the risk of getting cancer.'

The chapter explains the classic experiment by Tversky and Kahneman, who first found that gain-framed and loss-framed messages have different persuasive effects. Since then, however, research has shown prospect theory is too simple to explain message framing effects. The chapter discusses three of the most studied factors that influence the effects of gain- versus loss-framed messages. These are:

1 the perceived 'riskiness' of the target behaviour through the eyes of the audience;
2 their self-efficacy (or confidence) in relation to performing the behaviour;
3 the extent to which a 'fit' is established between the message frame and the receiver.

Conclusions and recommendations

The way in which each factor affects interpretation of loss- versus gain-framed messages is explained and advice is given on how to choose gain or loss frames in messages. The authors advise using a loss frame if performing the behaviour is perceived to be risky by the target audience and readers are likely to have high confidence in their ability to perform the behaviour.

The chapter concludes that gain frames generally are the 'safe' option for health promotion text design.

11.10 Summary of Chapter 10 Computer-tailoring of health promotion messages

In this chapter, Johannes Brug and Anke Oenema describe computer-tailoring. This involves using an instrument such as a survey to measure a range of characteristics, beliefs and behaviours and then allowing a computer program to provide individualised health promotion messages that are matched to each recipient's responses. Previous chapters have recommended that messages should be tailored to the knowledge and concerns of the target audience. The advantage of computer-tailoring is that messages can be tailored personally – to the individual recipient.

They describe how a computer-tailored intervention consists of the following components;

1   a theoretical framework which identifies what may need to be changed in order to promote the target behaviour;
2   a screening or diagnostic instrument that assesses each recipient in relation to a range of antecedents that may require change;
3   a database system that stores the individual responses;
4   a message library containing a range of messages;
5   a computer program that defines 'tailoring algorithms' to select the appropriate messages for any given response to the screening instrument;
6   a computerised format which can coherently deliver the selected messages to the respondent.

The authors present convincing evidence indicating that this approach to health promotion is more effective than generic health promotion (in which materials are written for large groups or populations).

This chapter also highlights how developments in web-based and phone-texting communication provide new opportunities for delivering personally tailored health promotion.

Writing health communication

11.11 Conclusion

We hope you will find, or have found, these chapters helpful in (1) deciding how to go about designing health promotion messages, (2) what to include in health promotion messages and (3) how to design and present such messages. In doing so we hope you will more effectively change people's health-related behaviours and so help them improve their health and well being.

Note

The work was partially supported by the National Institute for Health Research (NIHR) UK. However, the views expressed are those of the authors and not necessarily those of the NIHR or the UK Department of Health.

Index

NOTE: Page numbers in *italic type* refer to figures and tables.

Index

Index

observational data, 58
O'Connor, D.B., 138
online text *see* websites
open recall questions, 60
Orbell, S., 85
orientation of pages, 9
orphans in text, 12
outcomes measures, 122–3
overviews, 50

page orientation, 9
page sizes, 8–9
paging, 52, 61
Payne, S., 1
perception *see* risk perception; susceptibility
perceptual organisation, 53–4, 57, 68–9
personal relevance, 124–5, 128
    see also computer tailoring; susceptibility;
        tailored messages
personalisation of messages, 157
persuasion
    impact on self-efficacy, 91–2
    role of graphics, 71
    see also fear appeals; message framing
Peters, L.H.W, 101
Petty, R.E., 95
photographs, 72–3, 74–5
physiological reactions, impact on
        self-efficacy, 91
pilot studies *see* pre-testing
planned ignoring, *107*
planning
    of evaluations, 113–14
    goals and, *108*
    instructions prompting, 129–30
    of interventions, 100–1, 102–3
    model of, 146
point sizes, 15, 20
'point-of-choice' settings, 149
portrait orientation, 9
practice, to enhance self-efficacy, *106*
pre-testing, 5, 20, 65, 96, 114, 140
    for comprehension, 28, 36, 38, 39
    of computer tailored messages, 154–5
    and graphics, 36, 38, 81
    for usability, 58–61
    see also evaluation
precaution adoption process model (PAPM), 152
preparatory behaviours, 85–6
presentation *see* audience understanding;
    graphics; layout and typography; usability
prevention messages, framing, 136–7, 138, 140–1
printed computer tailoring, 154
prior knowledge, 26, 44–5, 64
process evaluations, 114
progressive muscle relaxation, *108*
promotion messages, framing, 140–1

Pronin, E., 137
prospect theory, 135–6, 137, 138
protection motivation theory, 126
proximity, of text and graphics, 31, 54, 78–9
pushbuttons, on websites, 55

questionnaires, 61, 151, 152

randomised controlled trials, 113–14, 122
readability measures, 60
readers *see* audience
reattribution of success/failure, *106*
Reit, J. Van 't, 140
response efficacy, 125–6, 127
reviews
    of goals, *108*
    see also evaluation
rewards, 95, *109*
risk
    explaining with graphics, 68, 78
    and message framing, 135–6
    see also fear appeals
risk assessment, 128
risk perception, *104*, 136–9
road safety, 119, *120*
role models, 91, *105–6*, 158
Rothman, A.J., 137

safe sex interventions, 92–3
    condom use promotion, 84–7, 88–9, 92, 93–6
    fear appeals, 119, *120*, 123–4
Salovey, P., 137, 138
samples, 58–9, 123
sans-serifs, 17–18
satisfaction, 44, 61
scanning, 43, 67
Schaalma, H., 112
Scheinberger-Olwig, R., 95
Schinke, S.P., 92
screening instrument, for computer
        tailoring, 151–2
scrolling, 52
search options, on web pages, 49
searching
    role of graphics, 67–8
    and testing for efficiency, 61
self reward, *109*
self talk, *107*
self-affirmation, *107*, 125
self-efficacy, 91–3, *94*, 96, 99, 112
    and fear appeals, 126, 127
    and message framing, 139–40
    techniques to enhance, *106–7*
self-image, 91, *93–4*
self-monitoring, *107*, 128
self-regulatory skills, 92
sequences, 75–7

serifs, 17–18
severity, and fear appeals, 125, 126, 127, 130–1
Sheeran, P., 85–6
similarity, 54
size
    of graphics, 72
    of pages, 8–10
    of type, 15–16, 20, 53–4
skills, 88, 90, 91, 92, 108–9
Small, J.P., 10
Smith, J., 4
smoking interventions
    and fear appeals, 118–19, 120–1, 122,
        124, 125
    help to stop, 128, *129*, 130
SMS (short text messaging), 158
Sobczyk, A., 103
social comparison, *105*
social identity, *105–6*
social pressure, 90–1, *93*, 95–6, *108–9*
    see also normative beliefs
social skills, 92, *108–9*
social support, *109*
spacing text, 10–15, 53, 54
spatial-contiguity effect, 32
stimulus control, *109*
stimulus-response compatability, 48–9, 55, 58
subjective evaluations, 58
subjective norm, 87
    see also normative beliefs
success, reattributing, *106*
sunscreen use, 137
support
    social support, *109*
    to stop smoking, 128, *129*, 130
susceptibility, perceptions of, 125, 126,
        127, 128
systematic processing, 95, 96

table of contents, 46, *47*, 52, 53–4, 58
tables, 68, *77*, 78
tabs, 49, 50, 56–8
tailored messages, 148–9
    see also computer tailoring
tailoring algorithms, 153–4
target group segmentation, 148
targeted health promotion, 148
technology, use in computer tailoring, 158
testing *see* evaluation; pre-testing
text
    advance organisers in, 29
    and comprehension, 24–8
    relationship with graphics, 31, 32, 54, 77,
        78–9, *80*, 118, 119

text messaging (SMS), 158
text processing, 44–6, 59
    see also attention processes; cognitive
        processing
text spacing, 10–15, 53, 54
text structure, 3
    and graphic organisers, 29–31
    and learnability, 51
    and perceptual organisation, 53–4
    role of spacing, 11–12
    understanding, 60–1
    and usability, 46
textual coherence, 26–8
textual health warnings, 118, 119, 121
theoretical models, 88–93, 90, 101, 110
    for computer tailored messages, 150–1, 152
theory of planned behaviour, 86, 90, 110, 152
theory of reasoned action, 86, 90
threat appraisal, 126, 139
tobacco products, 118–19, 120–1, 122, 125
    see also smoking interventions
top-down processing, 44–6
tree diagrams, 29–30
Tversky, A., 135–6
type-sizes, 15–16, 20, 53–4
typefaces, 16, 17–18
typographical design *see* layout and
        typography
typographical reference grid, 15

unjustified text, 12–13
US presidential election, 14
usability, 43–4, 62, 163
    applying criteria, 55–8
    criteria, 46–55
    and structure, 46
    testing for, 58–61
user guidance scheme, 54–5, 56, 57
users *see* audience

vertical lists, 19, 54
vertical spacing, 11–12, 13–15
visual attention, 59
visual grouping, 53–4, 68–9
volitional processes, 130
voting forms, 14

Walker, R.C., 14
web-based tailoring, 154, 158
websites, usability, 48, 49, 50, 51, 52, 53, 54, 55
weight loss interventions, 102–3, 134, 157
widows in text, 12
working memory (WM), 24, *25*, 32, 53, 54, 57
World Health Organization, 118

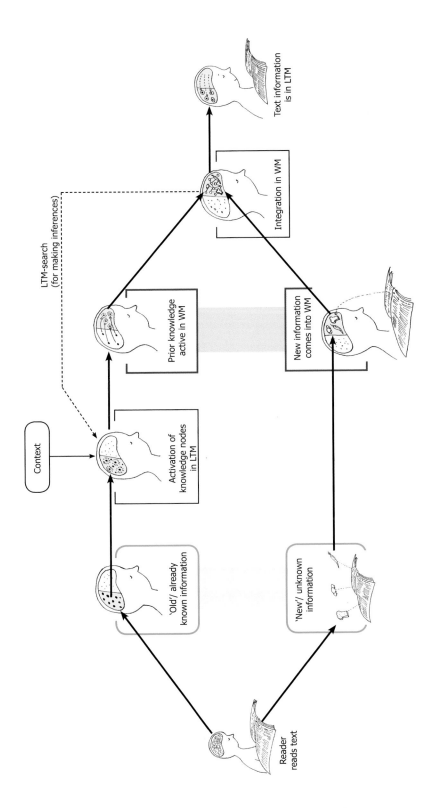

Figure 3.7 Adjusted version of Figure 3.1 Note how the use of illustrations make the rather abstract psychological explanations easier to envisage and therefore understand and memorise. The colours indicate which elements of the graphics are important and in combination with the slightly differently shaped surrounding lines they link different phases depicted in the graphic, with each other.

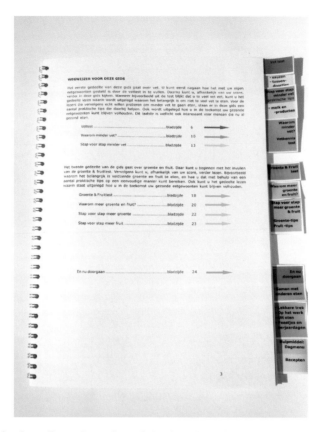

Figure 4.3(b)   An adjusted version of the brochure in Figure 4.3(a), adjusted according to the eight usability guidelines described in the text

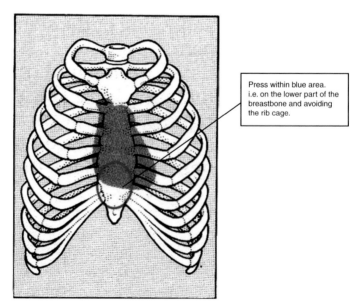

Press within blue area.
i.e. on the lower part of the
breastbone and avoiding
the rib cage.

Figure 5.5   Diagram with a blue oval indicating where to apply pressure during resuscitation

Source: Tony Smith (2000) *The British Medical Association Complete Family Health Encyclopedia*, p. 237.

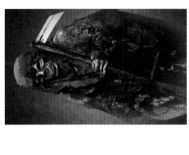

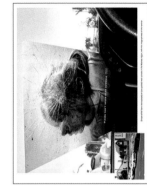

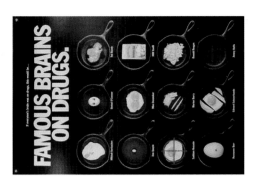

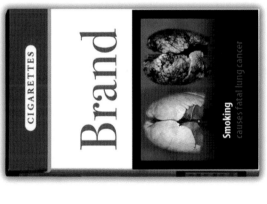

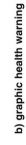

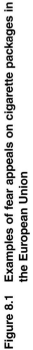

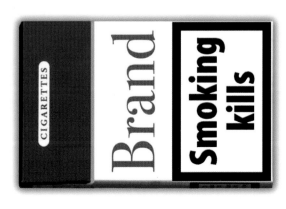

Figure 8.2 Further examples of fear appeal messages

© Environment Waikato. Available at: http://creativity-online.com/work/
environment-waikato-please-dont-speed/8968

© Australian Department of Health. Available at: http://www.avert.org/
media-gallery/image-236-the-grim-reaper-australia-aids-campaign-1987

© Capital Concepts, Inc

CIGARETTES

Brand

**Smoking
kills**

CIGARETTES

Brand

Smoking
causes fatal lung cancer

a) Textual healthwarning

b) graphic health warning

**Figure 8.1 Examples of fear appeals on cigarette packages in
the European Union**

© European Union

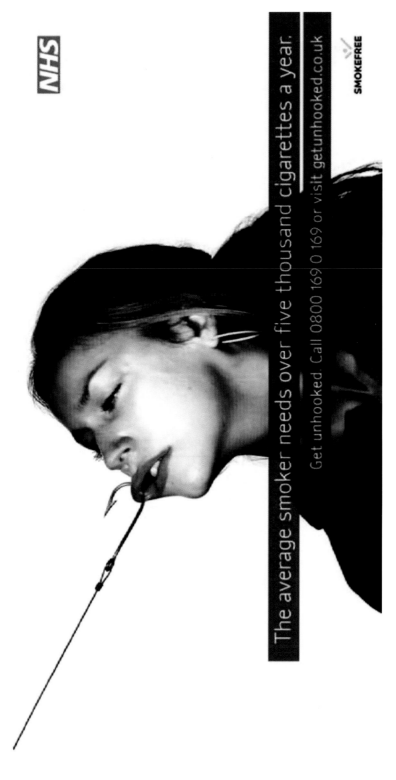

Figure 8.4 UK National Health Service; Anti Smoking 'Get Unhooked' advert Crown Copyright, Department of Health 2009, available at: http://smokefree.nhs.uk/resources/resources/product-list/detail.php?code=1724906340

© Crown copyright, Department of Health 2009, available at: http://smokefree.nhs.uk/resources/resources/product-list/detail.php?code=172496340